T0245290

DESIGNING EEG EXPERIMENTS FOR STUDYING THE BRAIN

ELSEVIER *science & technology books*

Companion Web Site:

https://www.elsevier.com/books-and-journals/book-companion/9780128111406

Designing EEG Experiments for Studying the Brain: Design Code and Example Datasets
Aamir Saeed Malik and Hafeez Ullah Amin

Resources available:

Table of Contents:
- Chapter Abstracts
- Chapter Data
- Glossary

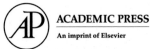

ACADEMIC PRESS
An imprint of Elsevier

DESIGNING EEG EXPERIMENTS FOR STUDYING THE BRAIN

Design Code and Example Datasets

AAMIR SAEED MALIK

HAFEEZ ULLAH AMIN
Universiti Teknologi PETRONAS, Perak, Malaysia

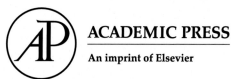

ACADEMIC PRESS

An imprint of Elsevier

Academic Press is an imprint of Elsevier
125 London Wall, London EC2Y 5AS, United Kingdom
525 B Street, Suite 1800, San Diego, CA 92101-4495, United States
50 Hampshire Street, 5th Floor, Cambridge, MA 02139, United States
The Boulevard, Langford Lane, Kidlington, Oxford OX5 1GB, United Kingdom

Copyright © 2017 Elsevier Inc. All rights reserved.

No part of this publication may be reproduced or transmitted in any form or by any means, electronic
or mechanical, including photocopying, recording, or any information storage and retrieval system,
without permission in writing from the publisher. Details on how to seek permission, further
information about the Publisher's permissions policies and our arrangements with organizations such
as the Copyright Clearance Center and the Copyright Licensing Agency, can be found at our website:
www.elsevier.com/permissions.

This book and the individual contributions contained in it are protected under copyright by the
Publisher (other than as may be noted herein).

Notices
Knowledge and best practice in this field are constantly changing. As new research and experience
broaden our understanding, changes in research methods, professional practices, or medical treatment
may become necessary.

Practitioners and researchers must always rely on their own experience and knowledge in evaluating
and using any information, methods, compounds, or experiments described herein. In using such
information or methods they should be mindful of their own safety and the safety of others, including
parties for whom they have a professional responsibility.

To the fullest extent of the law, neither the Publisher nor the authors, contributors, or editors, assume
any liability for any injury and/or damage to persons or property as a matter of products liability,
negligence or otherwise, or from any use or operation of any methods, products, instructions, or ideas
contained in the material herein.

British Library Cataloguing-in-Publication Data
A catalogue record for this book is available from the British Library

Library of Congress Cataloging-in-Publication Data
A catalog record for this book is available from the Library of Congress

ISBN: 978-0-12-811140-6

For Information on all Academic Press publications
visit our website at https://www.elsevier.com/books-and-journals

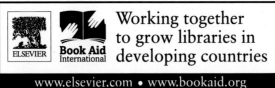

Working together
to grow libraries in
developing countries

www.elsevier.com • www.bookaid.org

Publisher: Mica Haley
Acquisition Editor: Natalie Farra
Editorial Project Manager: Kristi Anderson
Production Project Manager: Kirsty Halterman and Karen East
Designer: Alan Studholme

Typeset by MPS Limited, Chennai, India

CONTENTS

LIST OF FIGURES

LIST OF TABLES

PREFACE

This book is intended for those who are planning brain studies using electroencephalography (EEG) as well as those who want to explore new clinical and behavioral applications using EEG. Prior knowledge of brain functionality and neuromodalities is required for understanding the material provided in this book. This book is not about EEG or about the brain; there are already large numbers of books available on such topics. Therefore, the reader may wish to go through the basics of brain anatomy and physiology as well as the basics of EEG before studying this book. Also, there are many good resources available on the Internet to study the basics of the brain and EEG.

This book is specifically beneficial for those who want to venture into this field by designing their own EEG experiments as well as those who are excited about neuroscience and want to explore various applications related to the brain. This book details experimental design for various brain-related applications like stress, epilepsy, etc., using EEG. The main aim of the book is to provide guidelines for designing an EEG experiment. As such, the first chapter provides details on how to design an EEG experiment as well as the various parameters that should be considered for a successful design. Chapter emphasis is on ethical issues, sample size computation, and data acquisition guidelines. An example of stimulus experiment design is also provided. Various types of EEG equipment and software are also discussed in Chapter 1, Designing an EEG Experiment.

The remaining 13 chapters provide experiment design for a number of applications including clinical as well as behavioral applications. In addition, experiment design codes and example datasets for one subject are provided with each chapter. As each of the chapters is accompanied by experiment design codes and example datasets, those interested can quickly design their own experiments or use the current experiment design for their own experiments. The appendices provide various forms, including a recruitment form, feedback form, and various forms for the subjective tests associated with the chapters. Also the chapters provide recommendations for the related hardware equipment and software for data acquisition as well as processing and analysis.

Chapter 2, Mental Stress; Chapter 3, Major Depressive Disorder; Chapter 4, Epileptic Seizures; Chapter 5, Alcohol Addiction; Chapter 6, Passive Polarized and Active Shutter 3D TVs; Chapter 7, 2D and 3D Educational Contents; Chapter 8, Visual and Cognitive Fatigue during Learning; Chapter 9, 3D Video Games; Chapter 10, Visually Induced Motion Sickness; Chapter 11, Mobile Phone Calls; Chapter 12, Drivers' Cognitive Distraction; Chapter 13, Drivers' Drowsiness; Chapter 14, Working Memory and Attention are each organized similarly. In general, they start with the introduction of the problem being discussed in the chapter, followed by the specific problem statement and the objectives of the study. After that, details are provided for the hardware and software used in that specific study. The experiment design and protocol section includes target population, sample size computation, inclusion and exclusion criteria, experiment design, and experiment procedure. Then the data description is provided and the details of the data accompanying the chapter are discussed. Finally, relevant papers and references are given.

Two chapters are provided where the experiment design for studying stress and depression are discussed in detail, i.e., Chapter 2, Mental Stress, on stress and Chapter 3, Major Depressive Disorder, on major depressive disorder (MDD). The stress experiments involve designing stimulus experiments for studying four levels of stress. This is done through using various stimuli to induce the stress and then measuring the corresponding brain signal using EEG. Chapter 3, Major Depressive Disorder, provides details on the experiment that can be used for both diagnosis of MDD and monitoring the treatment efficacy of antidepressants for MDD patients.

Chapter 4, Epileptic Seizures discusses the issue of epilepsy. Because a large population is affected by epileptic seizures, the related researchers' motivation is to come up with new methods that can diagnose as well as predict the onset of epileptic seizures. Chapter 4, Epileptic Seizures, provides details on epilepsy and discusses various datasets that are available for studying epilepsy. One of them is from MIT in the United States while the other two datasets are from Europe. Chapter 5, Alcohol Addiction, details an experiment for objectively recognizing alcohol use disorder (AUD) patients. AUD subjects are classified into two categories, i.e., alcohol abuse (AA) and alcohol dependent (AD). Both AA and AD are described distinctly according to the *Diagnostic and Statistical Manual of Mental Disorders IV (DSM-IV)*, as a severe form of alcohol drinking that causes distress or harm to the drinker. In this chapter, EEG data collection for discriminating AUD from control and for discriminating AA and AD is discussed.

Chapter 6, Passive Polarized and Active Shutter 3D TVs; Chapter 7, 2D and 3D Educational Contents; Chapter 8, Visual and Cognitive Fatigue during Learning; Chapter 9, 3D Video Games; Chapter 10, Visually Induced Motion Sickness are related to various aspects of multimedia. Chapter 6, Passive Polarized and Active Shutter 3D TVs, looks at the two three-dimensional (3D) consumer electronics display technologies, i.e., active shuttered and passive polarized based displays. An experiment is designed to study which one of these technologies is superior when compared with traditional two-dimensional (2D) displays. This is done by using videos of various 3D movies as the stimulus for the experiment. Chapter 7, 2D and 3D Educational Contents and Chapter 8, Visual and Cognitive Fatigue during Learning are related to learning using the various types of multimedia tools. An experiment design is provided to compare learning with 3D tools compared to traditional 2D tools. In addition, as learning is related to memory, the design of the stimuli includes experiments for studying both short-term and the long-term memory. Chapter 8, Visual and Cognitive Fatigue during Learning uses the event-related potentials (ERPs) extracted from the EEG signal to study visual and cognitive fatigue during learning. This is important as many studies have reported that fatigue due to 3D multimedia tools can affect the memory retention process.

Chapter 9, 3D Video Games, uses 2D and 3D games as stimuli to study two things: the differences in brain activity for each of the gaming modes (2D and 3D) that result in different experiences for the subject, and the effect of violent games on subjects' brain activity. Hence, the experiment discussed in this chapter addresses two different questions. Chapter 10, Visually Induced Motion Sickness is important as it provides an experiment design to study visually induced motion sickness (VIMS). VIMS has been reported in the form of nausea, headache, disorientation, and discomfort after watching 3D movies and after playing 3D games. Hence, a special movie is designed as stimulus to induce VIMS in the subjects.

Mobile phones have become a part of our daily lives and are one of the most important technical gadgets that we carry with us all the time. A number of studies have reported contradictory findings about the effects of mobile phone usage on our brain. Chapter 11, Mobile Phone Calls, provides details of an experiment that was conducted to study the effects of mobile phones using EEG. The experiment involves four conditions, two with the right ear and two with the left ear. One of the conditions involves touching the ear while the other involves answering the phone without touching the ear by keeping it at a certain distance from the ear.

Chapter 12, Drivers' Cognitive Distraction, and Chapter 13, Drivers' Drowsiness, deal with another important aspect of our lives: driving. Almost everyone is exposed to driving in one way or another. We are either driving ourselves or traveling in a vehicle driven by others. It has been reported in many transport safety-related reports that the majority of accidents are due to the driver. Hence, in these two chapters, an experiment design is provided for studying two important parameters related to driving, i.e., driver cognitive distraction and driver drowsiness. The stimulus for studying cognitive distraction involves asking the subject to answer analytical and logical questions while driving. For driver drowsiness, the subject drives on a long road with monotonous environment for a long time, and EEG signals are recorded while the subject drives.

Finally, Chapter 14, Working Memory and Attention, is related to working memory and attention. There are three processes related to memory, i.e., memory formation, memory retention, and retrieval. The experiment in the chapter specifically addresses the memory formation and maintenance stages. Attention, distraction, and interruption are used in the stimuli to study the memory stages.

After the design of experiments and collection of data, the next stage is the preprocessing, processing, and analysis of the EEG data. We plan to publish another book that will explain the process of analysis of EEG data for the various brain-related applications mentioned in this book. In the meantime, the readers can access the papers listed in the "Relevant Papers" section in each of the chapters. These papers provide the details of various analysis techniques for particular applications. In the upcoming book, a step-by-step guide will be presented to analyze the data, and complete details of the analysis techniques with MATLAB code will be provided.

CHAPTER 1

Designing an EEG Experiment

Contents

Designing EEG Experiments for Studying the Brain.
DOI: http://dx.doi.org/10.1016/B978-0-12-811140-6.00001-1

© 2017 Elsevier Inc.
All rights reserved.

1.1 INTRODUCTION

Electroencephalography (EEG) is a reliable and widely used measurement tool for studying brain functions, abnormalities, and neurophysiological dynamics due to its low cost, noninvasiveness, portability, and high temporal resolution in the millisecond range.[1] In the field of neural signal processing, EEG is commonly used as a noninvasive brain imaging technique for diagnosis of brain disorders and normal EEG for understanding of brain functions in research studies. It enables the researchers and clinicians to study brain functions such as memory, vision, intelligence, motor imagery, emotion, perception, and recognition, as well as detect abnormalities such as epilepsy, stroke, dementia, sleep disorders, depression, and trauma. EEG signals reflect the electrical neuronal activity of the brain, which contains useful information about the brain state. This chapter will discuss the fundamentals of EEG, EEG experiments, ethical approval guidelines, sample size computation, experiment design, EEG equipment and presentation software, and EEG data acquisition.

1.2 FUNDAMENTAL OF EEG WAVES

Since the beginnings of EEG, the study of different brain oscillations and their relationship with different brain functions has attracted the attention of researchers. Hans Berger discovered the presence of alpha and beta waves in EEG. The brain oscillations are categorized in frequency bands and related with different brain states or functions. In this section, a brief description of EEG frequency bands is provided. A typical example of EEG waves can be seen in Fig. 1.1.

1.2.1 Delta Waves (Up to 4 Hz)

EEG delta waves are high-amplitude brain waves and are associated with deep sleep stages. The delta waves are also associated with different brain functions other than deep sleep, e.g., high frontal delta waves in awake subjects are associated with cortical plasticity. Delta bands are reported as prominent brain waves in cognitive processing especially in event-related studies.[2] EEG low-frequency components, especially delta bands, are the primary contributor to the P300 peak of event-related potentials (ERPs). P300 is a widely studied and well-known indicator of cognitive processing.

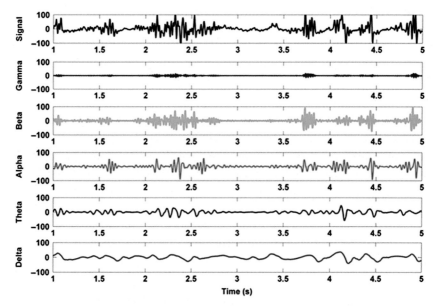

Figure 1.1 EEG signal and corresponding bands.

1.2.2 Theta Waves (4–8 Hz)

Theta waves are observed in the drowsy state and more common in children than adults. In the awake adult, without doing any attention/cognitive activity, high theta activity is considered abnormal and associated with different brain disorders, e.g., high frontal theta is linked with nonresponse to antidepressant treatment in depression patients. However, high theta activity plays a significant role in attentional processing and working memory, see for review.[3] Changes in theta activity are also reported in brain disorders such as depression in adults and dyslexia in children. Pizzagalli et al.[4] reported that better responders to treatment in major depressive disorder (MDD) showed high theta activity in the rostral interior cingulate (BA 24/32). Klimesch et al.[5] reported reduced theta activity in dyslexic children.

1.2.3 Alpha Waves (8–13 Hz)

Alpha waves can be observed spontaneously in normal adults during wakefulness and in relaxed state, especially when there is no mental activity. During the eyes-closed condition, alpha waves are prominent at parietal locations. Attentional processing or cognitive tasks attenuate the alpha waves. Alpha waves are subdivided into lower alpha and upper alpha. It has been observed that alpha activity changes with load during retention of working memory.[6] In addition, individual alpha peak frequency is an indicator of general intelligence factor (also known as *g* factor).[7]

1.2.4 Beta Waves (13–25 Hz)

Beta waves have lower amplitudes than alpha, delta, and theta waves. Traditionally, beta waves are subdivided into low beta and high beta. The frontal and central regions of the brain are locations where enhanced beta waves can be observed during activeness, anxious thinking, problem solving, and deep concentration. Gola et al.[8] reported that beta band power is increased over occipital sites during spatial discrimination tasks and visual attention in high-performing participants both young and aged. A detailed review on beta band activity is provided by Engel and Fries[9] where evidence is given about beta activity involvement in cognitive processing and the motor system.

1.2.5 Gamma Waves (above 25 Hz)

Gamma waves are fast oscillations and are usually found during conscious perception. Due to small amplitude and high contamination by muscle artifacts, gamma waves are underestimated and not widely studied as compared to other slow brain waves. High gamma activity at temporal locations is associated with memory processes. Research studies reported that gamma activity is involved in attention, working memory, and long-term memory processes (see Ref. 10 for review). Gamma activity is also involved in psychiatric disorders such as schizophrenia, hallucination, Alzheimer's disease, and epilepsy (see Herrmann and Demiralp review[11]).

1.3 IMPORTANCE OF EXPERIMENT DESIGN

Every scientific research study starts with a question and ends with a possible solution. In experimental research, especially in brain research, the question may be as general as "what brain regions are associated with the state of depression and stress?" or "what is the role of alpha band in stress and anxiety?" The experimental question pushes the researchers to derive a research hypothesis, which is a description about how a given manipulation can change certain measurements. The research hypothesis may be general or specific, like a research question. An example of research hypothesis in EEG research is the statement, "EEG alpha activity at frontal cortex will be reduced in depression patients." In a hypothesis statement, the researchers can make particular claims, such as, "EEG frontal alpha activation in right frontal region will be high compared to left frontal lobe." The scientific characteristic of a hypothesis is that it should be tested experimentally. Highly specific hypotheses can be easily falsified and are more informative.

To test a hypothesis, a researcher or experimenter designs an experiment. In experiments, first manipulate some aspect of the research problem and then measure the outcome of that manipulation; e.g., Galileo's experiment of the effects of mass on gravity. He speculated that an object's acceleration due to gravity is independent of its mass. He tested this hypothesis by dropping two balls of different masses from a certain height and observed that they fell at an equal rate. In this procedure, first he manipulated the mass of the objects being dropped and then measured the time required for the balls to fall from a given height. The manner in which a researcher organizes the manipulations and measurements of an experiment is the experimental design. The required skills for experimental design may differ from one discipline to another; however, in this chapter the focus is on EEG experiment design.

In general, every researcher wants to investigate their research question about the world and design an experiment to find a meaningful solution to this research question in the most efficient way. Thus, the experiment needs to be designed well in each and every aspect.

In EEG research, significant resources are required in terms of equipment cost, time, and human resources (including experimenters, subjects, and research assistants). The EEG setup procedure normally takes 20–30 minutes; data collection sessions vary widely depending on the number of trials or conditions. Typical EEG experiments have up to 20 participants per condition or group of interest.[12] The number of participants varies based on the size of the effect to be tested and the number of trials to be collected per participants. In addition, the raw EEG requires human efforts to clean the unwanted artifacts present in the signal. Therefore, an inadequate EEG experiment design will create great trouble to the researchers, because it will either fail to answer the defined hypothesis or provide results that are hard to interpret to make a conclusion. Thus, all the investments in the form of time and money would be wasted. The researchers are required to make a good plan and consider each and every step of the experiment from participant recruitment to interpretation of the final results, including all the possible risks, restrictions, confounding variables, and resources. The characteristics of well-designed experiments are as follows[13–15]:

- as simple as possible to operate for the experimenter and easy to reproduce for later researchers
- tests a specific hypothesis and provides fair estimates of the factor effects and associated risks
- minimum cost of running experiment and enables experimenter to detect significant differences
- includes planning for data analysis and results interpretation
- allows to make conclusions that have wide validity

These characteristics are very general; each researcher is required to look the associated different parameters with respect to the research problem and the available resources in order to make a well-designed EEG experiment. For particular guidelines for subject preparation in EEG and ERP experiments with human participants, see the work of Light and colleagues.[12]

1.4 EEG EXPERIMENTATION: ETHICAL ISSUES AND GUIDELINES

Experimentation on animal and human subjects has a long history in scientific and medical literature. It is essential for scientific progress and the promotion of medical well-being to use human subjects during experimentation. However, research risks are always there and unavoidable. Therefore, the use of human subjects in experimentation especially in health care generates ethical, legal, political, and humanistic concerns. Although in the literature, no severe health-related issues have been reported in noninvasive scalp EEG recordings, there are still many concerns that need to be considered in EEG experiments on human subjects.

1.4.1 Ethical Issues

The most important issue is the subject's informed consent, i.e., whether the subjects are competent to decide on their participation. This is especially serious when children, patients, or disabled subjects are involved in studies. What should be included in the informed consent? Sometimes the information provided in the informed consent is not sufficient. The lack of knowledge of the subjects about the experiment may mislead them to be incompetent for the experiment.

1.4.2 Ethics Approval Guidelines

The following are general guidelines to be considered in EEG research for ethics approval.

1.4.2.1 General Principles

- The responsibility of the ethics committee is to ensure ethical standards of experimental research, protect the rights, dignity, and well-being of human participants, and defend the researchers from unfair criticism. In addition, the ethics committee also ensures the benefits of the study to society. Thus, every EEG experiment involving human participants must go through ethics review and ethical approval by a standard authorized ethics committee before initiation of the experiment.
- In case EEG experimentations need to be undertaken in another institution or outside the university, where a local ethics committee is available, then it is the responsibility of the researcher to obtain the approval of the local ethics committee.
- The researchers must design such an experiment to ensure that the research study will benefit society and they should follow sound principles throughout the experimentation.
- It is the responsibility of the principal investigator to ensure that there is no conflict of interest in the proposed experimental work, including publication, ownership of the data, subsequent use of the data, and sources of funding. The conflict of interest may be personal, academic, institutional, or commercial.

1.4.2.2 Participants' Rights

- Each and every participant has the right not to participate in the experiment, and the researcher must respect this right. University staff, students, and any other human with dependent relationship must be assured that any decision to refuse participation will not affect their academic/employment progress.
- All the participants should be protected from mental, psychological, physical, social, and legal risks throughout the experimentation. In case of any aftereffects, the participant should have proper information and full contact details as to whom they should contact including neurosurgeons, as well as a psychiatric or at least general physician. All the research staff and participants must be fully aware of any potential hazardous or uncomfortable contexts expected during the experiment.

- Each participant has the right to withdraw from the experiment without any reason or penalty.
- Participants have the right to any question, and they must be assured that their privacy and identity will be protected.

1.4.2.3 Informed Consent

- The aim of the informed consent is to arrange experiments openly and transparently without any fraud. Therefore, the participants must be provided full information about the research experiments as much as possible to make it clear for the participants or their parent/guardian, if children are subjects, to decide their involvement.
- The informed consent must contain clear explanation of EEG to be used during data collection, and ensure health and safety concerns.
- All the research staff to be involved in experimentations must be aware about the protocol of the experiment and its potential risks.
- The informed consent should be given on a written consent form along with a separate participant information sheet. The signature of the participant must be taken before the start of the experiment. In case the participants are not able to give informed consent or are under the age of consent, then consent must be obtained from the parent/guardian. The ethics committee should have written principles about the consent of children and/or disabled participants.
- The consent form must contain a clear description about sharing the research data, publication of results, and reuse of data at a later stage. The details of privacy and confidentiality procedures should be clear to the participant about the data management including accessing, storing, and usage.
- The researcher should provide a copy of the signed consent form to the concerned participant.

1.4.2.4 Participant Recruitment and Remuneration

- The recruitment of human participants for experimental work through advertisements, e.g., social websites, university portals, or any other digital media, should be included in the ethics approval and require permission of ethics committee.
- The researchers should clearly advise the participants, in advance, about any financial benefits, e.g., time compensation, expenses, or loss of wages. However, any incentives to be paid to the participants in terms of money require approval from the ethics committee.

1.4.2.5 Ethical Principles of Related External Bodies

- The researchers must follow the university ethical guidelines along with any external governing body controlling or monitoring the universities, e.g., the Ministry of Education and Health & Medical Council.
- If the experimentations are to be conducted with partner or collaborator institutions other than the researchers' host university, then the researchers must consider any ethics procedures and regulatory principles of the partners' or collaborators' institutions.

1.5 SAMPLE SIZE COMPUTATION

Sample size computation is an important aspect of neuroscience, behavioral, and clinical investigations. Practically, it is not feasible to include the whole population in any research study. There is always a common question, "how many individuals should be included in the research study?" Thus a small set of individuals is selected from the population that is small in size but statistically sufficient to represent the target population. Empirically, the goal is to make inferences about a population from a sample. There is no fixed number of sample size for a certain study. However, in practice, sample size is determined based on the expense of data collection and should be large enough to have sufficient statistical power. Here, general guidelines for sample size computation are given that will help the researchers in clinical studies as well as in related disciplines to understand clearly the prerequisites and to compute sample size.

1.5.1 Objective and Hypothesis of the Study

It is critical that the objective and hypothesis of the study are clear before determining sample size calculation. What does the researcher want to investigate? Well-defined objectives will lead the researchers to extract relevant information from prior studies to be used in sample size calculation, e.g., mean differences, variance, standard deviation, and effect size. These parameters are normally required to be used as input in the formulas or software for sample size calculation.

1.5.2 Target Population

Target population is the entire group of people or animals or objects to which the researcher wants to generalize the findings of the experiment, e.g., all females with major depression disorder, all children below 10 years with a learning disability, all males above 65 years with dementia. Target population should be well-known and access to the individuals in the target population should be planned. If the population is spatially widespread and not easily accessible, it may cost a great deal to collect data with a large sample size.

1.5.3 Statistical Attributes of Sample Size

There are a few important statistical parameters in calculating sample size, such as statistical power, significance level, effect size, and standard deviation. The statistical power and significance level are fixed by convention, but the effect size and standard deviation need to be computed from previous studies. These parameters are described in the following subsections.

1.5.3.1 Statistical Power

The statistical power (sensitivity) is the probability that a statistical test will detect a difference when a true difference exists. In other words, it is the probability of correctly rejecting a false null hypothesis. In experimental studies, sometimes the researchers fail to detect a difference when actually there is a difference (false negative). This false negative rate is referred in statistics by the letter β and known as type-II error. Statistically, power is equal to $1 - \beta$. If the power of an experimental study is low, then there is a chance that the study will fail to detect true difference. The acceptable figure of power in statistics is 80%. However, above 80% power is a good study design.

1.5.3.2 Significance Level

The significance level (α level) is the criterion used for rejecting a null hypothesis when it is true. The α value is normally set to 5% (0.05). For example, it is acceptable that the probability that the result observed due to chance (not due to experimental intervention) is 5%. In other words, the acceptable detection of a difference is 5 out of 100 times when actually no difference exists (false positive or type-I error).

1.5.3.3 Effect Size

Effect size is the difference between the value of the variable in the intervention group and control group. J. Cohen (1988) suggested that the effect size (referred to as d) be considered small, medium, and large if $d = 0.2$, 0.5, and 0.8, respectively.[16] This implies that if the mean difference of two groups or conditions is less than 0.2 standard deviations, then the difference will be trivial even if it is statistically significant. The effect size is normally based on previously reported studies and has high influence on sample size value. If the effect size is large between the study groups then a small sample is required to detect the difference and if the effect size between the study groups is small, then a large sample size is needed to find the difference.

1.5.3.4 Standard Deviation

Standard deviation tells about the distribution of data. It is denoted by Greek letter sigma (σ). The value of sigma is generally adopted from previous studies' findings and used in sample size calculation. If the data is normally distributed, then about 68% of the data points lie within one standard deviation, about 95% are within two standard deviations, and about 99.7% lie within three standard deviations.

1.5.4 Types and Numbers of Dependent and Independent Variables

The researchers should define the dependent variable (DV) and independent variable (IV) and their types involved in any study. The IV is the experimental variable, which is intentionally manipulated and hypothesized by the investigator to test the cause and effect in the DV. In an EEG/fMRI (functional magnetic resonance imaging) experiment, the IV can be a stimulus (e.g., three-dimensional (3D) image), task (oddball), age, or gender. In clinical trials, the IV can be a placebo, new medicine, neurofeedback therapy, antidepressant, or antiepileptic drugs (AEDs). The DV is the quantifiable variable measured by the investigator to find the effect of the IV. An example of DV in the case of an fMRI experiment can be BOLD signal in a certain region of brain. In the case of an EEG experiment, DV can be theta power, peak alpha power, and peak frequency. In an ERP experiment, DV can be P300 amplitude or latency, N170, and late positive or negative component. The type of DV is important to be known, and it can be quantitative, or qualitative. In EEG experiments, the DV type is always quantitative.

1.5.5 Groups, Conditions, and Statistical Tests

The number of groups or conditions involved in any study should be identified by the researcher. The identification of groups or conditions will help the researchers to decide which statistical test should be adopted for analysis. If only one group is involved in the study and two conditions (pre- and postintervention) are under investigation, then the investigation will be within subjects and a paired t-test can be a suitable statistical test to be applied during analysis. In case a study is between subjects, then there will be two groups involved, e.g., healthy versus control. In this case, the IV is the different populations of subjects and an independent *t*-test can be applied during analysis. Having more than two groups or conditions in any study demands an advanced statistical test such as analysis of variance (ANOVA), and repeated measures ANOVA. For detailed understanding of statistical tests, any resource of statistics can be consulted, e.g., Dupont WD. *Statistical Modeling for Biomedical Researchers: A Simple Introduction to the Analysis of Complex Data*. Cambridge University Press, 2009.

1.5.6 Available Software

Many online resources including websites, books, and programs provide principles for sample size computation using various techniques. There are software programs developed for determining the sample size for clinical research studies. A few of them are described here.

Power Analysis and Sample Size (PASS) software provides tools for sample size computation, over 680 statistical tests, and confident interval scenarios. Each tool is validated with published research work. The detail and trial version can be downloaded from the website (http://www.ncss.com/software/pass/).

Power and Sample Size (PS) is a free program for performing sample size calculation in continuous, survival response, and dichotomous measures. The PS software can work on both windows and Linux/Mac operating systems. In addition, it can explore the relationship between power, sample size, and detectable alternative hypothesis. Free download of PS version 3.2.1., 2014 is available at http://biostat.mc.vanderbilt.edu/wiki/Main/PowerSampleSize.

Biomath (http://www.biomath.info/power/index.htm) is an online program from the Division of Biostatistics, Columbia University Medical Center that can compute sample size. The program has a simple interface that asks about the number of groups and type of statistical test to be used in the study. After selecting the number of groups (one group or two groups) and statistical test, on the next page it will require the mean difference and standard deviation (if one group and paired t-test were previously selected). The mean difference and standard deviation information will come from previously conducted similar studies. In special cases, when the mean difference and standard deviation from the literature is unavailable, then sample size may be selected without computation by an expert and the research study will be a pilot study.

HyperStat is online statistics book (http://davidmlane.com/hyperstat/power.html) that provides discussion of statistical parameters, including sample size computation, with links to access-related resources such as statistical tests.

1.6 EXAMPLE OF EXPERIMENT DESIGN

Experiment design is the process where the stimuli are defined and it is decided how to present the stimuli to the participants. This can be done using a variety of presentation software. One of most popular presentation software packages is E-Prime. In this section, an experiment design example of an oddball paradigm, a well-known ERP task, is explained step by step using E-Prime software. Each step and structure of program is described here. The complete experiment file of the oddball task can be found in the bookData\chap01.

1.6.1 Objective

Before starting any experiment design in any presentation software, it is necessary that the objective of the experiment is clearly defined. The objective of the experiment in fact fulfills the objective of the study. The researcher should answer such related questions before starting the experiment: who are the target participants? (human, animal, young, old, children, male, female, healthy, patient etc.); which mental process is under study? (working memory, decision making, reasoning, intelligence, information processing, visual response etc.); how and which brain region is the responder? (left frontal in depression, central parietal for alpha peak, left temporal in memory retrieval etc.); and which brain modality is to be used? (EEG, fMRI, fNIR, MEG, etc.). Once the objective of the experiment is known then the rest of the steps are easy to complete.

Example:

Who are the target participants?

Answer: Healthy university graduates with age between 18 and 30 years.

Which mental process is under study?

Answer: Visual P300 component (amplitude and latency).

How and which brain region is the responder?

Answer: In visual stimulus task of ERP, the central parietal site is the best responder to the P300 component.

Which brain modality is to be used?
Answer: EEG 128-channel device will be used to map the brain activity.

1.6.2 Instructions to Participant

In each and every experiment, it is important to define the instructions to the participant in an understandable manner. The instructions may vary from task to task and depend on the target participants. When the researcher finalizes the target participants, the instructions will be prepared accordingly.

Example: Welcome and Instructions Screen in Oddball Task
Welcome to the Oddball Experiment
   You will see on screen a Box or Sphere
   The Box will appear frequently
   You have to Press '0' when you see the Sphere, otherwise do nothing.
   Press SPACEBAR to Start session!

1.6.3 Stimulus and Time

The type of stimulus should be defined (e.g., visual, or auditory) and the researcher should design the stimulus to induce the expected changes in the neuronal system of brain that is hypothesized in the study.

Example: There are two visual stimuli (Fig. 1.2); one is a 3D box and one is a 3D sphere. The duration of visual stimulus presentation is 500 ms on screen to the participant. The reason for keeping the duration to 500 ms is that the visual information can reach the occipital lobe within 100 ms in healthy adults' brains. The parietal lobe can respond around 300 ms after the onset of stimulus.[17]

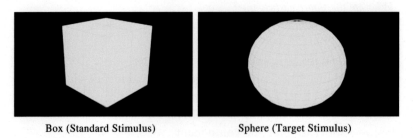

   Box (Standard Stimulus)   Sphere (Target Stimulus)

Figure 1.2 Example of visual stimulus in oddball task.

1.6.4 Trials, Blocks, and Conditions

The number of trials of each stimulus and total number of trials should be specifically defined in the design. If there are different conditions involved then the number of blocks can be more than one, e.g., if practice trials are required to be presented to the participants then a separate block for practice can be defined. In Fig. 1.3, the structure of the oddball task is shown using E-Prime. There is a "SessionProc," which is a main component of every E-Prime based experiment. The "SessionProc" object contains "instructions screen," "goodbye screen," and two components of the Net Station software package, i.e., "NSinit" and "NSUnint." Net Station is data acquisition software for the EGI EEG systems. The Net Station software package helps the E-Prime software to communicate with the Net Station (data acquisition software). The purpose and functions of each of these components are described below.

- "NSinit": To initiate EEG recording and confirm the interfacing between E-Prime and Net Station. When the "NSinit" command is executed during running the experiment, a few milliseconds EEG recording is initiated in the data acquisition software (Net Station). This will happen when E-Prime is properly connected with the Net Station software and the EGI EEG equipment is properly configured. Running E-Prime without the connection to Net Station and the EEG equipment will give a warning/error; see Fig. 1.4. In designing

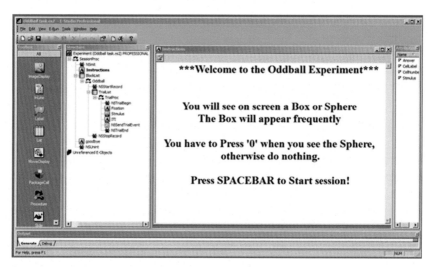

Figure 1.3 Structure of oddball task in E-Prime software.

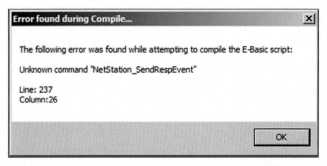

Figure 1.4 Error message when E-Prime is not connected with Net Station while Net Station package is added.

a new experiment, the Net Station package should be added at the final stage after the confirmation of instructions, stimulus, trials, blocks, feedback, and final "goodbye" statement.

In the case of an already-designed experiment like in this example, if E-Prime is required to run without EEG recording to test the experiment, the Net Station components can be easily removed by right clicking and pressing delete.

- "NSStartRecord":This command tells Net Station to start EEG recording.
- "NSTrialBegin":This command informs Net Station about the beginning of a trial.
- "NSTrialEnd": This command informs Net Station about the ending of a trial.
- "NSStopRecord": This command instructs Net Station to stop the EEG recording.
- "NSUnint": This command will close the communications between Net Station and E-Prime.

In the second level of hierarchy in the oddball experiment structure, there is a "BlockList" object. In the "BlockList" all the blocks of the experiment can be listed. Here, in the oddball experiment, only one block is added, i.e., the "Oddball" block. In the block of "Oddball," there are two Net Station objects, "*NSStartRecord*" and "*NSStopRecord,*" and one "TrialList" object. As there are two types of stimuli involved in the experiment (standard and target stimuli), each stimulus needs a separate trial along with other attributes to be explicitly defined in the object "TrialList"; see Fig. 1.5. The weight of the standard stimulus is 95 and weight of the target stimulus is 40, which is an approximately 70/30 ratio. The "Nested" attribute is empty, because there are no subtrials inside the standard or target trials.

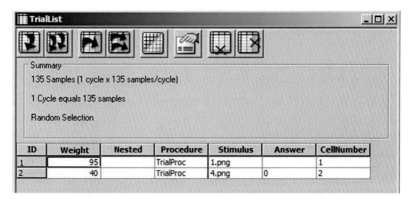

Figure 1.5 Triallist of oddball experiment.

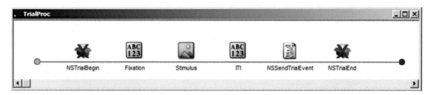

Figure 1.6 Objects of TrialProc.

The "Procedure" attribute defined the actual procedure name "TrialProc" to be executed 95 times for standard stimulus and 40 times for target stimulus. The "Stimulus" attribute defined the actual names of the stimuli, which are 1.png and 4.png. The "Answer" attribute defined the actual response against each stimulus. As on the instructions screen, it is mentioned that only target trials (sphere stimulus) need subjects' response (pressing the 0 button). Therefore, in the "Answer" attribute, only target trials are defined with a "0" value. In the "CellNumber" attribute, the standard and target trials are assigned a unique identifier. This identifier can be used in Net Station to analyze EEG data, especially in segmentation of trials.

Inside the "TrialProc" object, the actual events include fixation, stimulus, ITI (intertrial interval), script (NSSendTrialEvent), and two Net Station objects, "*NSTrialBegin*" and "*NSTrialEnd*"; see Fig. 1.6.

1.6.5 Participants' Response and Feedback

In general, EEG experiments consist of participant responses against the stimuli where they mentally (e.g., counting the occurrence of certain stimuli) or physically do any action like pressing a button. E-Prime allows recording of these responses by creating a data file each time the E-Prime experiment is executed and completed. The researcher needs to set the parameters, such as setting a certain keyboard or mouse button, reaction time, and response accuracy, that are desired to be recorded in E-Prime at the stimulus property menu; see Fig. 1.7. A tag (stm+) can be added to the stimulus in the "common" tab, so that when a stimulus appears during the experiment, EEG recording will be stamped with a "stm+" tag. Stimulus background can be set in the "general" tab in the stimulus property, i.e., the duration of stimulus, input device such as keyboard, allowable key to be pressed, action on stimulus once the participant respond, and data logging (by default is the standard option).

In the tab "Duration/Input," the correct answer is set to "Answer," which is the attribute of target trials defined in "TrialList"; see Fig. 1.7. Here, in the stimulus property, the stimulus is bonded with the trials and the allowable keyboard key is to be used as the participant's response.

Some experimental tasks need to provide feedback to participants during the running of the experiment, e.g., informing the participant about the accuracy of the response. For this purpose, E-Prime provides a "feedback display" object that can be linked with participant response and can

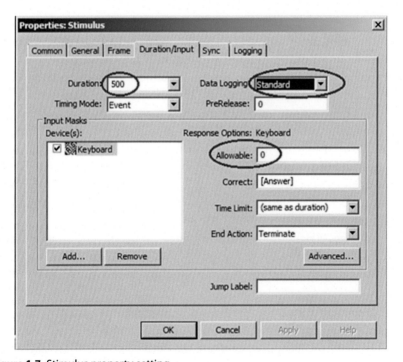

Figure 1.7 Stimulus property setting.

be displayed on the screen immediately after recording the participant's response. In this oddball task example, there is no feedback screen.

1.6.6 Events Synchronization with EEG

To stamp certain events on EEG recordings, E-Prime provides a programming option to synchronize events such as fixation onset, stimulus onset, stimulus, offset, subjects' responses, and trials information.

Example: The following code will send fixation and stimulus information including trials information, onset, offset, and subjects' responses. To gain more expertise in E-Prime programming, the E-Prime manual can be consulted (https://www.pstnet.com/).

```
'Send response event using data collected from specified object
NetStation_SendRespEvent c, Stimulus
'Send a trial event for each presentation in the trial
NetStation_SendTrialEvent c, Fixation
NetStation_SendTrialEvent c, Stimulus
'Send the trial specific event
NetStation_SendTRSPEvent c, Stimulus
```

1.6.7 End of Task

At the end of each experiment, the participant is informed about the completion of the experiment and given further instruction (if any); otherwise, a thank-you message is displayed on the screen as shown:

```
***The oddball task is ended. ***
    Thank-you very much for your participation!
```

1.7 EEG EQUIPMENT AND SOFTWARE

1.7.1 EEG Equipment and Data Acquisition Software

EEG data acquisition is a time-consuming activity that needs clear objectives and proper planning to acquire the desired EEG signals. In the market, various manufacturers provide various EEG devices from low density to high density, dry electrodes and gel-based electrodes, wire and wireless amplifiers, along with acquisition software with different features other than data recordings. In this section, a list of some of the available EEG devices is provided with brief details and distinct features (see Table 1.1).

Table 1.1 Detail of EEG devices and manufacturers

Equipment	Description
EGI EEG	Electrical Geodesics, Inc. (EGI) offers EEG technology for neuroscience research with easy-to-use Geodesic Sensor Net 32, 64, 128, and 256 sensor nets that incorporate with analysis software. The data acquisition software is called Net Station and offers interfacing with stimulus presentation software, records the subjects' details, and records EEG data. The Net Station software allows analysis of the raw EEG and extracts ERP signals. Raw EEG can be exported to other formats such as .mat files and .edf files (https://www.egi.com/).
BrainMaster EEG	BrainMaster Technologies, Inc. has developed a 24-channel EEG and a DC amplifier that is an evolution of the technology, called Discovery 24E. The Discovery 24E offers a next generation qEEG and EEG biofeedback system that is both high quality and low cost for research communities. The Discovery 24E consists of low-noise DC sensitive amplifiers, 24-bit analog-to-digital converters, and optically and magnetically isolated USB interface. The 24 channels include 22 channels dedicated for EEG, plus 2 channels of differential inputs with separate references. The data acquisition software is known as Discovery, and is capable of interfacing with stimulus presentation software, recording participants' information, and recording and saving EEG data.
MITSAR EEG	MITSAR Co. Ltd has developed EEG systems including 21 channels, 24 channels, 31 channels, and 48 channels. MITSAR allows a maximum sampling rate of 2000 Hz and AD conversion 16 bit to 24 bit. Data acquisition and data analysis software are included in the package (EEGStudio and WinEEG). WinEEG includes filtering, montages, wavelet and spectral analysis, 3D mapping, spike detection, dipole source localization, ERP signal analysis, importing and exporting data. For more details, visit http://www.mitsar-medical.com.
Enobio EEG	Neuroelectrics offers wireless multichannel EEG and transcranial current stimulation such as tDCS, known as Enobio and Starstim, respectively. The EEG Enobio systems include Enobio 8, Enobio 20, and Enobio 32-channel devices. The data acquisition software is known as Neuroelectrics Instrument Controller (NIC). NIC can be used for both Enobio EEG systems as well as Starstim devices. NIC can work on both Mac and Windows platforms. For more detail about data acquisition with Enobio systems using NIC software, please visit http://www.neuroelectrics.com/products/enobio.

(*Continued*)

Table 1.1 Detail of EEG devices and manufacturers (Continued)

Equipment	Description
Emotiv EEG	Emotiv has developed a wireless 14-channel EEG EPOC system for brain control interfacing and EEG data. The system includes 14 sensors for EEG recording and 2 references. Sensors need electrolyte solution to get better conductivity and strong EEG signal but no skin preparation is needed. The EPOC system works with a chargeable battery that can be continuously used for 12 hours if charged fully. The EPOC system works with a USB dongle to communicate with EPOC control panel/testBench software for data storage and controlling BCI devices. For further details, visit https://emotiv.com.
CADWELL Arc EEG	Cadwell Industries, Inc. manufactures medical devices including an EEG system, called Arc Essentia. It is a 32-channel EEG amplifier with 7 active and reference pairs with 250–500 Hz sampling rate. The data acquisition software of Arc Essentia is capable of video recording, acquisition control, spike detection, and auto achieve. For more details, please visit, https://www.cadwell.com/arc.
EGOSPORT EEG	ANT-Neuro has designed the compact eego sports 64-channel amplifier with complete freedom to collect high-density EEG, bipolar EMG signals, and a variety of physiological sensor data. It also works with a battery for up to 6 hours of recording. The amplifier is directly connected with the tablet and data transfer does not depend on the quality of wifi or Bluetooth connection. The data acquisition software (eego software) provides a friendly user interface, managing new and existing subject entries, guiding users through setting up new recordings, and reviewing data files. Other features are basic filtering, artifact correction, averaging in time and frequency domain, and advanced signal processing methods such as 3D mapping and source reconstruction. For further details about data acquisition with eego sports, visit https://www.ant-neuro.com/products/eego_sports.
BIOSEMI	BioSemi provides various medical instrumentation including EEG devices. The BioSemi EEG (Active Two System) consists of 280 active channels with DC amplifier and 24-bit resolution for research applications. It provides from 2 to 16 kHz/channel sampling rate, which is adjustable. For more detail about the features of the system, visit http://www.biosemi.com/products.htm. The data acquisition software is based on the LabView programming language. The software can handle basic functions such as data acquisition, display data on screen with scaling and filtering options, network sharing, and storing data in .BDF file format. In addition, the BioSemi hardware system can interface with well-known EEG software such as BESA and Neuroguide.

(Continued)

Table 1.1 Detail of EEG devices and manufacturers (Continued)

Equipment	Description
NeuroScan	NeuroScan provides a variety of EEG acquisition systems and analyses of ERP data such as SynAmps RT, Grael, Siesta, and NuAmps amplifiers. The SynAmps RT EEG system provides 64-, 128-, and 256-channel amplifiers including unipolar and bipolar electrode configurations. The Grael system is capable of recording 32 channels for EEG with 8 bipolar and 8 high-level inputs. The NuAmps is a high quality and low cost 40-channel EEG amplifier that is capable of 22-bit sampling at 1000 Hz. The Siesta is a 32-channel wireless EEG amplifier. It allows the subject to move during recording and can record EEG data. The sampling rate is 1024 and bit resolution is 16. Curry 7 Suite is the data acquisition software and is capable of online processing of EEG/ERP data, including signal processing and basic source analysis. The complete details for NeuroScan systems can be found on their website: http://compumedicsneuroscan.com.
BIOPAC	BIOPAC Systems, Inc. offers a 32-channel wireless EEG amplifier Mobile with high-fidelity wireless EEG data with water electrodes. The bit resolution is 24 and the range of wireless recording is 10 m indoors. The channels are unipolar and the data acquisition software AcqKnowledge is easily configured to create unique montages and combinations of signals. The device contains a trigger channel that can be used to synchronize EEG with subjects' responses against the stimuli in experiments. Further details are available at http://www.biopac.com/product/mobita-32-channel-wireless-eeg-system/.

1.7.2 Presentation Software

EEG recordings in an experimental environment during a certain cognitive task require stimuli that can induce changes in the neuronal networks that are under investigation. The stimulus may be visual or auditory depending on the aim of the research but in either case the synchronization of stimulus presentation with the induced neuronal activation is compulsory. This synchronization demands full control on stimulus manipulation in the experimental task. We have listed well-known stimulus presentation software available for fulfilling the requirements of researchers in Table 1.2.

Table 1.2 Stimulus presentation software

Software	Description
E-Prime 2.0	E-Prime is software designed to fulfill the computerized experimental need of researchers working in psychology, neurosciences, and biomedical areas. Presently E-Prime is being used in more than 5000 institutions in 60 countries. It provides a friendly environment in which to design simple to complex experiments and can be used by novices and advanced users as well. The E-Prime suites consist of E-Studio, E-Basic, E-Run, E-Merge, E-DataAid, and E-Recovery. All these packages enable the user to design experiments via drag-and-drop graphical interface, program in the scripting language, save data files, merge single-subject data files for group analysis, and perform data filtering, editing, analysis, and recovery of corrupted files. There is a long list of features including variety of stimulus support, interfacing with external devices, installation options, and experiment design. It is compatible with Windows and requires minimum dual-core 2 GHz with 1GB RAM, DirectX, and USB port. For more details about working in E-Prime, see the documentation and tutorial at https://www.pstnet.com/.
Inquisit	Millisecond Software was founded in 1999 by Sean Draine in Seattle, Washington. Millisecond provides Inquisit for psychological testing. The applications of Inquisit are clinical trials, cognitive and behavioral neuroscience, behavioral economics, decision making, human–computer interaction, sports, and psychology. A typical experiment designed in Inquisit consists of a single script file, plus any sporting media files, such as image, video, or sound, that are to be presented in the experiment as a stimuli. The structure of the scripting file of the experiment defines the components such as stimuli, trials, blocks of trials, and pages of instructions for the user, as well as the interaction of these components. The Inquisit programming has two simple syntactic constructions: elements and attributes. Each element has set of attributes that determine how that element behaves and corresponds to a component of the experiment (blocks, trials, stimuli). For details on experiment design in Inquisit, browse the manuals available at http://www.millisecond.com/support/docs/.

(Continued)

Table 1.2 Stimulus presentation software (Continued)

Software	Description
Presentation	Presentation is software for the display and arrangement of the stimulus in experiments for neuroscience. It can work on Windows and uses standard PC hardware. It was designed for behavioral and physiological experimentations that collect fMRI, ERP, EEG, and MEG data. Some of the main features of Presentation are multitasking, visual (including 3D images) and auditory stimuli control, eye tracker interfacing, synchronization with fMRI, programmability, and interfacing with external software such as MATLAB. To learn about experiment design with Presentation, see the tutorials available online at https://www.neurobs.com/presentation/docs/index_html.
Paradigm	Paradigm is software for stimulus presentation and control. The building blocks of Paradigm (Trials, Blocks, and Stimulus) are the same as other experiment design software. However, it allows designing experiments for mobile applications. It gives access to trigger commands through its Python scripting interface. The trigger accuracy is in milliseconds with EEG/EMG or TMS devices. It allows using USB port to parallel port. The programming guidelines and documentation about experiment design are available online at http://www.paradigmexperiments.com/Support/Docs/.
SuperLab	SuperLab software is designed for researchers, not for programmers. Its cross-platform allows use on either Mac or Windows. It supports many stimulus types such as pictures, movies, text, sound, rapid serial visual presentation (RSVP), and self-paced reading. Many other features include randomization, looping, feedback, stimulus lists, and contingencies. It supports input devices including keyboard, mouse, touch screen, microphone, RB series, lumina, SV-1 and PST serial response box. For more details about experiment design in SuperLab, see the manual available online at http://cedrus.com/superlab/manual/.
PsychoPy	This is an open-source application designed for stimulus presentation and data collection for wide range of neuroscience and psychology experimental research. It is free and is more powerful than other alternative software such as Presentation or E-Prime. It combines the graphical features of OpenGL with Python to give scientists a free and simple solution to stimulus presentation and control application. Since the software is open-source, it is easily modifiable. The advantages of using PsychoPy are platform independence, precise timing, multimonitor support, automatic monitor calibration, variety of stimuli, and simple installation. For more details on building experiments, see the documentation available online at http://www.psychopy.org/documentation.html.

1.8 GUIDELINES FOR EEG DATA ACQUISITION

EEG data acquisition is a fundamental and important activity of EEG-based research as the findings of experimental studies are highly dependent on the quality of data. In addition, if the intention is to record EEG during certain cognitive tasks such as working memory test then the experiment design plays a critical role. To ensure high quality of EEG data, the following guidelines need to be taken into consideration.

1.8.1 General Data Acquisition Setup

The general acquisition setup should be planned and previous literature should be consulted. The important factors are the number of EEG channels and their configuration (montage, bipolar, or referential), EEG reference selection, sampling rate, filtering, and recording of supplementary data.

1.8.1.1 Number of Electrodes

The main advantage of the EEG technique is the temporal resolution on millisecond scale as compared to other noninvasive brain mapping techniques such as fMRI. It is obvious that in multichannel EEG recordings, a certain number of electrodes are used for data acquisition, e.g., the standard international 10–20 system has 19 electrodes. However, a common question that may arise is, how many electrodes are needed? Should low-density EEG (such as 8 electrodes, 16 electrodes, or 24 electrodes) be used or high-density EEG (such as 64, 128, 256, and 512 electrodes)? The answer may depend on the objectives of the experiment, type of task to be performed, and the nature of the cognitive process to be investigated. Nevertheless, there are pros and cons of using either few electrodes or maximum electrodes. A high-density EEG system improves the spatial resolution but may take more time during setup. If the number of channels is 21 then a standard 10–20 montage can be selected.

- Dense electrodes create the opportunity for both biological artifacts (eye movement, blinks) and nonbiological artifacts (electromagnetic interference).
- Most EEG systems use electrolyte conductivity material; this electrolyte material may spread to the neighboring electrodes in the case of high-density EEG recordings.
- Low-density EEG requires less time to setup the electrode cap and reduce the impedance of the electrodes while high-density EEG systems need more time to set the electrode cap for recordings.

- High-density array EEG provides small interelectrode distance, which is highly recommended for highly localized signal sources.
- High-density EEG has high spatial resolution along with high temporal resolution. It means that more data will be acquired, which will definitely require large storage media, faster processing, and efficient memory chips, consequently resulting in greater expense compared to low-density EEG systems.

It is noted that the low-density EEG systems are easy in operations but not recommended for exploration of brain functions and source localization. In this context, a few studies have highlighted the issue of number of electrodes to be used in EEG recording for a certain purpose; e.g., Lantz et al.[18] investigated source localization for epileptic patients with different number of electrodes, i.e., 31, 63, and 123, and concluded that 123 electrodes would constitute a significant enhancement on the localization accuracy for epileptic patients.

1.8.1.2 Dry or Gel-Based Electrodes

EEG electrodes can be made of a variety of materials such as gold, silver, stainless steel, tin, and Ag/AgCl. The most widely used electrode material is Ag/AgCl, which provides low dc offset, establishes quickly and maintains stable electrochemical potentials, is free from allergenic compounds, and has long-term electrical stability. The electrodes may be active or passive. The electrode materials are the responsibility of the manufacturer of the EEG machines, to provide electrodes of suitable material such as Ag/AgCl. However, some manufacturers provide both gel-based (wet) and dry electrode options with EEG machines such as Enobio Starstim. The gel-based electrodes in general take more time to setup and the participants are required to wash their hair after EEG recordings because of the gel. However, once the gel-based EEG cap is set it will allow recording of good quality EEG for longer duration as compared to dry electrodes. The dry electrodes are very easy to setup as there is no need for gel or any electrolyte for good conductivity. However, the dry electrodes sometimes compromise the quality of the EEG and the patients/participants may feel irritation due to itching on the scalp because the dry electrodes need to be tightly attached to the scalp. Further, some dry electrodes have pin-like combs that may penetrate the scalp if used for longer durations of EEG recording. The dry electrodes have potential in brain–computer interface (BCI) applications.

1.8.1.3 Montage (Bipolar, Referential)

Montage is a combination of EEG electrodes during recordings. There are two main types of montage, i.e., bipolar and referential montages. In bipolar montage, two electrodes are required per channel, i.e., there is a separate reference electrode for each channel and no electrode is used as reference. However, the referential montage uses a single electrode as reference for all the channels, e.g., Cz as reference. The discussion on references is given in the following subsection. The most common referential montage is the international 10–20 system, which needs 21 electrodes. This 10–20 system is based on the relationship between the cerebral cortex and the location of electrodes over the scalp. The "10" and "20" come from the distance between the adjacent electrodes, which is either 10% or 20% of the total distance of the skull from nasion (front) to inion (back). Another common referential montage is the 10–10 system, which is an extension of the 10–20 system for high-density EEG recordings. The maximum number of electrodes in the 10–10 system is 81. However, as of 2016, 128-channel and 256-channel EEG systems are also available so the 10–5 system will allow the use of up to 300 electrodes; see Ref. 19 for details about these different systems.

1.8.1.4 EEG References

The EEG reference selection is a critical choice; the choice of reference may differ depending on the purpose of recording. There are many reference selection options such as earlobes, nose, mastoids, Cz, reference electrode standardization technique (REST), and averaged reference. Each reference type has its own advantages and limitations. It is recommended that researchers understand the background of these available reference options and choose the one most suited to their needs. It is to be noted that offline EEG data can be rereferenced; e.g., if Cz is used during recording then the offline data can be referenced to average reference or any other. Studies examining the comparison of different reference types have reported that averaged reference (AR) provides better results in separation of responders and nonresponders to treatment of MDD patients.[20]

1.8.1.5 Sampling Rate

The sampling rate is the number of quantitative values to be recorded in each channel per second such as 128 samples per second. The higher the sampling rate, the higher the temporal resolution of EEG recordings.

However, a very high sampling rate, like 2k per second, will require large storage media, system memory, and CPU processing. High sampling may be suitable for short-time EEG recordings such as time-locked EEG for the oddball task or any other cognitive task that includes trials of short-time period. As the brain processes the information very fast, changes can occur in microseconds. Therefore, when EEG is recorded with high sampling rate, it will allow analyzing the brain within microseconds. Furthermore, other parameters in EEG recording such as filtering should be defined and supplementary data such as electrocardiogram (ECG), electrooculogram (EOG), eye tracking, and video recording can be recorded, if required.

1.8.2 Experiment Design

The experiment to be used during EEG recording should be properly designed. For example in an event-related EEG experiment, there should be a sufficient number of trials to get the averaged signals after rejection of artifacts. The experiment should follow the ethical guidelines to ensure the participants' privacy, participants' consent, duration of experiment, instructions to participants, health-related risks, and the interventions, which induce the hypothesized changes in the brain. In case a participant does not feel comfortable during recording he/she may be disturbed and may engage in irrelevant movements, eye blinks, scratching, yawning, drowsiness, and loss of focus.

1.8.3 Preparation of Participant

The participant should be informed about the schedule of experimentation and the researcher should conduct the experiment to the ease of participants' availability. If the EEG device to be used in recording requires the participant to shampoo his/her hair, or avoid gel or lotion, then the researcher should ensure the participant's preparation accordingly prior to the experiment. If there are any other preconditions of the experiment such as proper sleep, avoiding drinks like coffee and alcohol, or physical exercise then the researcher should communicate with the participant to fulfill the preconditions. Prior to the start of the experiment, the participant should be well instructed about the experimental task and procedure of the experiment to avoid irrelevant movements, eye blinks/movements, and scratching during recordings.

1.8.4 EEG System Check-Up

To ensure the EEG equipment calibration, the instructions provided by the original equipment manufacturers (OEMs) should be followed. For the peripherals (such as electrodes/sensors), tuning the operation procedure of the equipment should be strictly followed to avoid calibration errors, and to utilize the sensors' full capacity of recording voltage potential.

1.9 SUMMARY

This chapter provides basics of EEG signal and different waves and their role in brain functions. Ethical and design issues of EEG experiments are highlighted. An important aspect of EEG research, sample size computation, is discussed and the factors that need to be considered in sample size computations are explored. Some sources of sample size computations are provided for beginners and intermediate researchers in EEG. An example of an EEG experiment using E-Prime with step by step guidelines is discussed. In addition, well-known EEG equipment and stimulus presentation software packages are listed with their key features. Guidelines are provided for EEG data acquisition and finally some general analysis of EEG is documented. All the material provided in this chapter may not be enough for each and every EEG experiment. However, the authors believe that this chapter will provide guidance to novice and intermediate researchers involved in EEG research in particular and biomedical engineering research in general.

REFERENCES

1. Haufe S, Nikulin VV, Müller K-R, Nolte G. A critical assessment of connectivity measures for EEG data: a simulation study. *Neuroimage*. 2013;64:120–133.
2. Amin HU, Malik AS, Ahmad RF, et al. Feature extraction and classification for EEG signals using wavelet transform and machine learning techniques. *Australas Phys Eng Sci Med*. 2015;38(1):139–149.
3. Amin H, Malik AS. Human memory retention and recall processes: a review of EEG and fMRI studies. *Neurosciences*. 2013;18(4):330–344.
4. Pizzagalli D, Pascual-Marqui RD, Nitschke JB, et al. Anterior cingulate activity as a predictor of degree of treatment response in major depression: evidence from brain electrical tomography analysis. *A J Psychiatry*. 2001;158(3):405–415.
5. Klimesch W, Doppelmayr M, Wimmer H, et al. Theta band power changes in normal and dyslexic children. *Clin Neurophysiol*. 2001;112(7):1174–1185.

6. Tuladhar AM, Huurne NT, Schoffelen JM, Maris E, Oostenveld R, Jensen O. Parieto-occipital sources account for the increase in alpha activity with working memory load. *Hum Brain Mapp.* 2007;28(8):785–792.

7. Grandy TH, Werkle-Bergner M, Chicherio C, Lövdén M, Schmiedek F, Lindenberger U. Individual alpha peak frequency is related to latent factors of general cognitive abilities. *Neuroimage.* 2013;79:10–18.

8. Gola M, Magnuski M, Szumska I, Wróbel A. EEG beta band activity is related to attention and attentional deficits in the visual performance of elderly subjects. *Int J Psychophysiol.* 2013;89(3):334–341.

9. Engel AK, Fries P. Beta-band oscillations—signalling the status quo? *Curr Opin Neurobiol.* 2010;20(2):156–165.

10. Jensen O, Kaiser J, Lachaux J-P. Human gamma-frequency oscillations associated with attention and memory. *Trends Neurosci.* 2007;30(7):317–324.

11. Herrmann CS, Demiralp T. Human EEG gamma oscillations in neuropsychiatric disorders. *Clin Neurophysiol.* 2005;116(12):2719–2733.

12. Light GA, Williams LE, Minow F, et al. Electroencephalography (EEG) and Event-Related Potentials (ERPs) with human participants. *Current protocols in neuroscience / editorial board, Jacqueline N. Crawley ... [et al]*; 2010;CHAPTER:Unit-6.2524.

13. Smith JA. *Qualitative Psychology: A Practical Guide to Research Methods.* London: Sage; 2007.

14. Carter M, Shieh JC. *Guide to Research Techniques in Neuroscience.* Burlington, MA: Academic Press; 2015.

15. Ward J. *The Student's Guide to Cognitive Neuroscience.* New York: Psychology Press; 2015.

16. Cohen J. *Statistical Power Analysis for the Behavioral Sciences.* Hillsdale, NJ: L. Erlbaum Associates; 1988.

17. Amin HU, Malik AS, Kamel N, Chooi W-T, Hussain M. P300 correlates with learning & memory abilities and fluid intelligence. *J NeuroEng Rehabil.* 2015;12(1):87.

18. Lantz G, Grave de Peralta R, Spinelli L, Seeck M, Michel CM. Epileptic source localization with high density EEG: how many electrodes are needed? *Clin Neurophysiol.* 2003;114(1):63–69.

19. Jurcak V, Tsuzuki D, Dan I. 10/20, 10/10, and 10/5 systems revisited: their validity as relative head-surface-based positioning systems. *Neuroimage.* 2007;34(4):1600–1611.

20. Mumtaz W, Malik AS, Ali SSA, Yasin MAM. A study to investigate different eeg reference choices in diagnosing major depressive disorder. *Paper presented at: Neural Information Processing*; 2015.

CHAPTER 2

Mental Stress

Contents

2.1 INTRODUCTION

Mental stress is defined as the reaction from calm to excited state for the sake of preserving integrity of the organism. Although stress study has been an active area in medical research since Selye first proposed it in 1936, it is not a universally accepted disorder.[1] This is because doctors tend to believe what they can perceive, read, or grade. The lack of measuring method for stress has kept it from being accepted in conventional clinical settings. On the other hand, human physiology has unveiled many facts about the variations in the human body, especially in the brain, that are caused by stress. These variations are measurable, detectable, and quantifiable through the application of neuroimaging techniques such as electroencephalography (EEG). EEG can record the changes in the neuronal networks due to stress or anxiety. Analysis of EEG using advanced signal processing methods such as discrete wavelet transform (DWT) can deal

Designing EEG Experiments for Studying the Brain.
DOI: http://dx.doi.org/10.1016/B978-0-12-811140-6.00002-3

© 2017 Elsevier Inc.
All rights reserved.

with the nonstationarity characteristic of EEG.[2] The variations in EEG thus can be detected and quantified to draw conclusions by using computational techniques.[3] The time-locked EEG can also be analyzed in a time domain to extract event-related potential (ERP) peaks to assess the effects of stress or mental fatigue.[4] This chapter provides details for the design of an experimental study that was conducted for exploring physiological stress patterns using time-locked EEG signals, and hence it serves as a guideline for those researchers and professionals who want to design EEG-based mental stress experimental studies.

2.2 IMPORTANCE OF MENTAL STRESS EVALUATION

Mental stress is a state of mind and does not have a physical existence, and is thus hard to describe. In addition, people handle their stress differently, i.e., some people are better at handling stress than others. However, there are many symptoms of mental stress explored during research studies as reported in the literature,[5,6] such as feelings of headache, tense muscles, low energy, upset stomach, nausea, chest pain, rapid heartbeat, and so on. The common concept of mental stress is a negative feeling, but stress may have good effects, e.g., it may push one to complete a task.[7,8] Stress affects many aspects of our lives including behaviors, mood, thinking, physical fitness, memory, and emotions. In situations where deadlines are required to meet with limited resources in a job environment, stress may be good[9]; however, long-term exposure to mental stress may lead to serious health issues.

Exact statistics on the number of people worldwide who suffer from mental stress disorder are not available. The reason may be that in most of the developing countries, people do not consider mental stress as an illness. Few health organizations in the United States and in developed countries have figures of mental stress disorders, e.g., according to American Psychological Association (APA) statistics from 2011, 53% of Americans reported personal health problems as a source of stress, 94% of adults believe that stress can contribute to the development of heart disease, depression, and obesity, but also 56% of adults reported that they are doing a good job of knowing when they are feeling stressed.[10] In the United Kingdom, the total number of cases of work–related stress, anxiety, or depression in the year 2014–15 was 440,000, i.e., a prevalence rate of 1380 per 100,000 workers.[11]

Clinicians and researchers have developed tools for mental stress assessment that are based on the feedback of the patients via Likert scale questionnaires such as perceived stress scale (PSS).[12,13] In such behavior-based stress assessment tools, the probability of finding the exact cause and impact of stress from the perception of the patients is low. Since mental stress is a psychological mental state, it would alter the normal neuronal activities of the brain. The assessment of stress via directly monitoring brain activities will enhance the diagnosis accuracy and help the clinicians to support their decision during treatment of patients about the severity of stress.

2.3 PROBLEM STATEMENT

Lack of objectivity in quantifying mental stress makes it an active research area. It has now been proven that mental alarm increases cognitive arousal and in turn results in cardiac variations.[14,15] The main research question that was addressed in this mental stress experimental study was "what is the quantitative difference between stress and control conditions?" The hypothetical statement of this study was that the mental stress affects heart rate and brain scalp potential. To investigate the heart rate and scalp potential, quantitative evaluation of electroencephalogram and electrocardiogram (ECG) signals were focused on in this study. These signals were recorded in a crossover experimental design where the participant performs a cognitive task in stress and control conditions. The following were the main objectives of this mental stress experimental study:
1. Finding the correlation between EEG and ECG measurements so that they will be effectively fused to increase the reliability of results.
2. Development of a novel scheme for the detection of mental stress.

The potential advantage of this experimental study is that it explores the brain dynamics accompanying cardiac variation; both can later be used to effectively detect mental stress.

2.4 SOFTWARE AND HARDWARE

In this experimental study, various software and hardware were used during data collection and analysis of data. All the experimental tasks were designed using E-Prime software, which was connected with the EGI Net Station data acquisition software during data collection to synchronize the events recording in E-Prime as well as in the EEG recordings. The EEG data was collected with EGI 128-sensor cap and ECG with two sensors connected to a polygraph. The EEG and ECG data can be exported to third party software such as MATLAB or Neuroguide for further analysis. EEG signals were preprocessed in EGI Net Station software and post-processed in Neuroguide software. The ECG signals were processed in MATLAB using Biosignal Toolbox.

The following software and hardware were used in this study for experiment design, data collection, and data analysis:

1. E-Prime 2.0 (for experiment design in how to present stimulus to the subject)
2. Electrical Geodesics, Inc. (128-channel EEG equipment with Net Station software)
3. MATLAB 2010 (for simulation)
4. Biosignal Toolbox
5. Neuroguide software
6. Statistical Package for Social Sciences (SPSS) for data analysis

E-Prime: E-Prime 2.0 is a psychology software for stimulus presentation in cognitive and behavioral research experiments (http://www.pstnet.com/eprime.cfm). This software is widely adopted in neuroscience research for stimulus presentation, control, and recording behavioral responses. It allows the users to control time synchronization of stimulus onset, offset, subjects' responses, and the corresponding EEG data. All the tasks used during this dataset are explained in the experimental design section. Details on each task in the E-Prime program are provided in the data description section.

EGI 300 amplifier & EEG nets: The hardware including the EEG nets and amplifier are from EGI Inc. (http://www.egi.com/). The EEG net contains 128 channels for recording of dense-array EEG from all over the scalp surface locations.

Net Station: Net Station is an EEG acquisition software that is used for recording EEG signals during learning and memory tasks. Net Station allows connection with the E-Prime software during running of the experiments for synchronization of time information for stimulus and subjects' responses. The raw EEG recording can be processed in Net Station, and includes processing operations such as filtering, segmentation, rereferencing, and exporting data to several other formats, e.g., .edf or .mat.

MATLAB: MATLAB is a high-performance programming language for technical computing and coding for engineering problems. It provides an integrative environment for use by engineers and scientists worldwide. The easy-to-use programming environment of MATLAB provides fast solutions to complex mathematical problems. The well-known disciplines of MATLAB programming are signal and image processing, communications and control systems, computational neuroscience and GUI programming, pattern recognition, and machine learning. For beginners in neuroscience, the book *MATLAB for Neuroscientists* by Pascal Wallisch and colleagues can be consulted.

BioSignal ToolBox: BioSignal ToolBox (http://biosig.sourceforge.net/help/index.html) is a collection of MATLAB functions for analysis of physiological signals including EEG and ECG.

Neuroguide: Neuroguide is EEG analysis software developed by Applied Neuroscience Inc. (http://www.appliedneuroscience.com/) in the United States. The software is well known for the analysis of qEEG data and generating participants' relative reports with respect to an EEG normative database.

Statistical Package for Social Sciences (SPSS): The SPSS was initially designed for social science problems by IBM. However, the software now includes many machine-learning algorithms such as clustering and classification. The SPSS is widely accepted for statistical analysis in disciplines including engineering and neuroscience.

2.5 EXPERIMENTAL DESIGN AND PROTOCOL

2.5.1 Target Population

The target population for this experimental study were the possible respondents that may meet the selected set of criteria and were available for the actual experiments. All the students in the university campus comprised the entire set of units for which the findings of the research had been generalized. Equal opportunity was given to all the students who met the inclusion criteria to become a participant.

2.5.2 Inclusion Criteria

The basic criteria necessary to be fulfilled by the potential participant in order to be a part of this experimental study are described as follows:
- Participant must be a student at Universiti Teknologi PETRONAS.
- Participant must be within the defined age limit (18–25 years).

- Participant must be physically and mentally healthy and must have never been diagnosed with any brain disorder in his/her medical history.

2.5.3 Exclusion Criteria

The exclusion criteria are the requirements used for the exclusion of participants from this study. The participants were excluded in this study when they:
- Failed to provide written consent.
- Failed to meet the requirements mentioned in the inclusion criteria.

2.5.4 Sample Size Calculation

The number of participants to be involved in the experimentation was determined by using the statistical methods based on previous studies. The actual sample size of 22 subjects was calculated to provide significant results from the experiment. The detail of the sample size calculation and corresponding information is given as follows:

Sample information: In this study, only one group of healthy persons was required.

Experiment conditions: There are two: one was control and other was stress condition.

Hypotheses: Both the null and alternative hypotheses are defined as following:
- *Null*: There is no change in heart rate, heart rate variability, and EEG signals during control and stress conditions.
- $\mu_{HR} \leq \mu_{oHR}$: The heart rate during stress condition is less than or equal to the heart rate in control condition.
- $\mu_{HRV} = \mu_{oHRV}$: Heart rate variability in stress condition increases or remains equal to heart rate variability in control condition.
- $\mu_{alpha} \geq \mu_{oalpha}$: EEG alpha power during stress condition is greater than or equal to that in control condition.
- *Alternate*: Control and stress conditions vary in heart rate, heart rate variability, and EEG signals.
- $\mu_{HR} > \mu_{oHR}$: The heart rate during stress condition is higher than in control condition.
- $\mu_{HRV} \neq \mu_{oHRV}$: Heart rate variability increases during stress condition.
- $\mu_{alpha} < \mu_{oalpha}$: EEG alpha power during stress condition is less than that in control condition.

Test criteria:

1. Significance level $\alpha = 0.05$ for 95% significance.
2. Power = 90% to reject null hypothesis, for that $\beta = 1 -$ power $= 0.1$.

The calculated number of participants to be included in the study was between 5 and 22. For sample size calculation, Power and Sample Size (PS) calculation software was used with paired t-test. The PS software is a free source for sample size computation developed by the Department of Biostatistics, Vanderbilt University (http://biostat.mc.vanderbilt.edu/wiki/Main/PowerSampleSize).

The formula for the sample size calculation is given below:

$$N = \frac{4(Z_\alpha + Z_\beta)^2 \sigma^2}{\delta^2} \tag{2.1}$$

where Z_α is the distribution of $\alpha = 1.642$ (for $\alpha = 0.05$); Z_β is the distribution of $\beta = 1.282$ (for $\beta = 0.1$).

2.5.5 Participant Selection and Recruitment

Standard procedure was followed to calculate sample size for the study followed by strict criteria to further shortlist the participants. A recruitment drive was done within Universiti Teknologi PETRONAS (UTP). Posters were displayed on notice boards on campus and in hostels for the announcement of subject recruitment for the experiment. All the students were encouraged to participate without any gender discrimination. Interested students were shortlisted based on the following criteria:

- They were all UTP registered students.
- The target age group was from 18 to 25 years old.
- Participants had no medical history of particular head injury or neurological disorders such as epilepsy, seizures, or migraine. They did not have skin allergies. They would also not be on daily medications that might alter the physiological data. This information was confirmed by using the Subject Recruitment Proforma Sheet (Appendix 2A).
- Shortlisted students were offered to fill out the PSS questionnaire (Appendix 2D) in order to further scrutinize the normal subjects (having no prior stress). PSS is a 10-question inventory that investigates how much an individual perceives stress in his/her personal life based on the experiences of the previous month. Every question is an experience in one's life that measures the strength with which situations are assessed as

stressful. Every experience or question can be scored from 0 (never) to 4 (very often). The scores for all questions accumulatively define a score that lies in one of four quartiles based on the severity of stress. These quartiles are 0–10, 11–14, 15–18, and 19–33[16] where the first quartile represents no stress and the last quartile represents the most severe stress. For the selection of subjects in this study, subjects falling in the last quartile were excluded as they were already under mental stress.

- Interested participants had to sign a consent form (Appendix 2C) after getting all the information about the experiment (see Appendix 14 for research information). They agreed that they willingly participated in the experiment and that they would appear in both sessions of the experiment.
- Based on these criteria, 22 subjects were selected, including two females. They had an average age of 22.54 ± 1.53 years. They were instructed not to take meals or energy drinks before coming to the experiment in order to avoid drowsy feelings or increased heart rate, respectively. They were also instructed to shampoo their hair to avoid recording of bad signals.

2.5.6 Experimental Design and Procedure

In order to record physiological signals, an experimental task was selected. The experimental task was an implementation of the Montreal Imaging Stress Task (MIST),[16] which had been designed for the purpose of inducing and processing mild psychological stress in terms of physiology and brain activation by using functional magnetic resonance imaging (fMRI). Fig. 2.1 provides an overview of the experiment flow. The experiment consisted of mental stress and control sessions, which took place on different days. The reason for selecting different days was first to minimize the learning effect,[17,18] so that at least a seven-day gap was given between the sessions,[18] and second to make the availability of subjects possible. A subject who appeared on one day might be available the next week on the same day.

The experimental procedure consisted of four sequential conditions: habituation, rest condition, mental arithmetic task (MAT) condition, and recovery condition. Both the sessions followed the same procedure except the MAT condition, which took place differently in both sessions. The core of the MAT was a computer-based arithmetic task followed by feedback on the response ("correct," "incorrect," or "no response"). However, under the stress condition, there was a time limit to solve the arithmetic task, along with distractions. Each of the MAT sessions lasted for 20 minutes. Moreover, to inspect gradual changes between stress and control conditions, the 20 minutes were divided into four equal intervals, which were

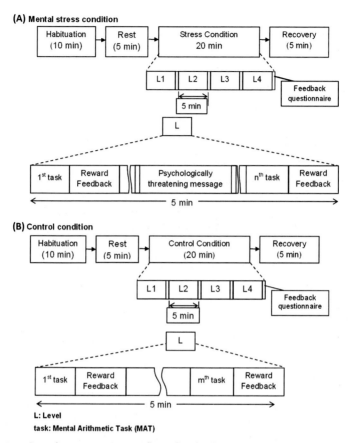

Figure 2.1 Complete experiment flow for both stress and control conditions. (A) Mental stress session. (B) Control session.

declared as four levels of the experiment. Each forthcoming level was of increasing difficulty. It should be noted that difficulty in a particular level was the same for both conditions. In order to eliminate the expected effect of conditions on results, half of the subjects performed the stress condition before the control condition and the other half of the subjects performed the control condition before the stress condition. All the tasks, experiment blocks, and conditions are discussed in the following subsections.

2.5.6.1 Habituation Period

The habituation period was designed to make the subject accustomed to the experimental environment. This included a rest of 5 minutes upon arrival. During this time, the subject was briefed about the experiment and was asked to provide written consent (for the consent form, see

Appendix 2C). Later, the subject was presented with tasks for 5 minutes for the following reasons:

- To solve sample questions of the actual arithmetic task.
- The answer to every trial was a single digit number (0–9), which required training to press the right key. The subject was presented with a single digit appearing on the screen and he/she had to press the same digit while looking at the screen to minimize eye movement.
- After the habituation period, the EEG and ECG sensors were put on the subject and recording of physiological signals was started.

2.5.6.2 Rest Condition

The rest condition was observed as the baseline for activations in stress and control conditions. The duration of this block was 5 minutes. Subjects were required to sit quietly with their hands lying on their thighs, open palms, upper teeth separated from lower teeth with the tongue floating inside the mouth, feet touching the floor, and legs not crossing each other. The subject needed to focus on a circle appearing on the computer screen in front of him/her. All these measures were taken in order to reduce the possibility of movement from the subject, so that unwanted artifacts might be reduced to a minimum.

2.5.6.3 Mental Arithmetic Condition

The MAT condition consisted of mental stress and control conditions, which took place in separate sessions, as shown in Fig. 2.1. Both the conditions were similar in the nature of the task, i.e., to solve arithmetic calculations. An arithmetic trial included up to four numbers (maximum 99) using four operands (addition (+), subtraction (−), multiplication (*), and division (/), e.g., $2 + 25/5$. Each condition had four levels, each of which lasted for 5 minutes. Experimental levels are described below.

Level 1

The tasks in level 1 required only two numbers under operations of addition or subtraction, e.g., $17 - 9$.

Level 2

In level 2, three numbers and an additional multiplication operator with addition or subtraction were used, e.g., $4 * 6 - 16$ or $3 + 2 * 2$.

Level 3

The tasks in level 3 needed four numbers and three possible operands (addition, subtraction, and multiplication) were used, e.g., $9 - 4 * 6 + 21$.

Level 4

Level 4 included four numbers including division, in addition to the other operations, e.g., $57/3 - 9 + 6$.

2.5.6.4 Stress Condition

The stress condition took place in the MAT condition in the session of mental stress. In this condition, mental stress was induced by the workload of arithmetic tasks and negative feedback.[19,20] Workload was created by offering limited time to solve arithmetic tasks. The duration of the trials at the four levels was 1200 ms, 3000 ms, 4000 ms, and 5000 ms, respectively. Along with the time limit in every trial, there was extra text ("delaying response text" and "speed up text") appearing with the stimulus on the screen to distract from the actual task and to induce more pressure on the subject. Fig. 2.2 displays a model of the computer screen. Text appearing on the screen is included in Table 2.1.

After every trial, along with the feedback on the response, the accuracy of correct responses and response time also appeared as reward. Moreover, after certain trials, a psychologically threatening message appeared on the

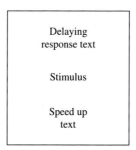

Figure 2.2 A model of the computer screen in the stress condition.

Table 2.1 Delaying response text and speed up texts to show on the screen

Type	Text	Level 1 (ms)	Level 2 (ms)	Level 3 (ms)	Level 4 (ms)
Delaying response text	Keep pace		Default		
	You are slowing down	1000	2000	3500	4000
Speed up text	Quick	700			
	Speed up		1000	1300	1200
	Faster		2000	2600	2500
	Hurry up			3500	
	Slow poke				3800

Table 2.2 A summary of stressful feedback messages

Level	Trial duration (ms)	Text feedback	Text
1	1200	After every 10 trials	Look at the screen and not at the keyboard. You are not following the instructions. You are slower in response than normal people. Be quick. Keep accuracy level 80%.
2	3000	After every 10 trials	Look at the screen and not at the keyboard. Be active in response. Sit attentively. This is the second level and still you are not familiar with the right keys. Give correct answers.
3	4000	After 10, 15, 20, 25, 30, 35, 40 trials	Don't guess answers. You are very sluggish in response. You have below average performance. How will you survive with this performance in next level.
4	5000	After 8, 15, 21, 25, 30, 34, 37 trials	Don't be overly smart. Don't guess answers. Don't leave questions unanswered. Money is subject to your performance. Your performance has been pathetic so far.

screen as negative feedback. This message was meant to portray the external pressures a worker would face in a work environment. The details of these feedback messages are provided in Table 2.2. This approach produced a high failure rate.

Before level 4 began, the experimenter reminded the subject that there was a required minimum performance level and that the subject's individual performance must be up to that level in order to include that subject's data in the study. Also the honorarium amount would reduce with wrong and unattempted questions. The subject was told about the need for standard performance across all subjects to allow the data to be grouped and would be reminded to press the correct key to submit their answer. Finally, the subject was told that his/her performance was under observation. This approach induced social stress in the subject.

2.5.6.5 Control Condition

The control condition took place in the MAT condition in the control session. For the control condition, the tasks were the same and equal in difficulty as the stress condition. However, there was no time restriction and no negative feedback in terms of psychologically threatening messages. The purpose of the control condition was to compare any cerebral activation caused by the mental arithmetic aspects of the task. Feedback ("correct" or "incorrect") would be displayed after each trial.

2.5.6.6 Recovery Condition

After the MAT condition was over, recovery time was given while the ECG and EEG details were recorded for 5 minutes. The recovery time was to find out what the changes were in terms of the signals when the subject was in the relaxed condition again.

2.6 DETAIL OF ETHICS APPROVAL

This research protocol was approved by the Ethics Coordination Committee of Universiti Teknologi PETRONAS and the Research Ethics Committee of Universiti Sains Malaysia.

2.7 DATA DESCRIPTION

The details of the EEG/ERP and behavioral data (subjects' responses) recorded during this experiment are provided below. In addition, the E-Prime stimulus design files for the stress and control conditions are also listed in Table 2.3.

2.7.1 Behavioral Data

Subject response (correct or incorrect or no response), reaction time (to answer the task), and subjective feedback (see Appendix 2B) were acquired after the experimental session was finished.

2.7.2 EEG/ERP Data

EEG raw data (nonaveraged), EEG artifacts free (averaged ERP data), E-Prime stimulus design files for control and stress conditions, behavioral responses, and event files for one subject are provided with this book. The details of these files are provided in Table 2.4. To access these files, please go to the directory BookData\Chap02 in the data files accompanying this book. For the complete dataset of 44 subjects (22 control and 22 stress), please contact the authors at brainexpbook@gmail.com.

Table 2.3 EEG/ERP data description

S. No.	File name	Description
01	Mental arithmetic task control condition S1_C_L1.edf S1_C_L2.edf S1_C_L3.edf S1_C_L4.edf C1.mat	This file contains the EEG data recorded while performing the mental arithmetic task during the control condition. In the control condition, there is no environment of stress. The file name contains L1, L2, L3, and L4, which presents the levels as mentioned in the experiment design section. This data is raw and nonaveraged (BookData\Chap02\ EEG Raw Data). All the events are embedded in the .edf files. The file "C1.mat" is an averaged clean data of the control condition that is extracted from the raw EEG data and then averaged over the trials. The "C1.mat" is a MATLAB array file containing the averaged data of all the four levels. The procedure of extracting trials from continuous EEG data to get averaged data is followed from Ref. 12. The clean data can be found in (BookData\ Chap02\ERP Averaged Data).
02	Mental arithmetic task stress condition S1_S_L1.edf S1_S_L2.edf S1_S_L3.edf S1_S_L4.edf S1.mat	This file contains the EEG data recorded during performing the mental arithmetic task during the stress condition. In the stress condition, there is an environment of stress induction. The participant has to solve the arithmetic task while stress is induced. These. edf files also contains raw EEG and nonaveraged data. The file "S1.mat" is the averaged clean data of stress condition that is extracted from the raw EEG data and then averaged over the trials. The file "S1.mat" is a MATLAB array file containing the averaged ERP data of all the four levels.

Table 2.4 E-Prime files of EEG stimulus experiment for stress and control conditions

S. No.	Experiment file name	Description
01	MIST_ control.es2	This file contains the experiment design for the control condition developed in E-Prime package E-Studio 2.0.
02	MIST_stress. es2	This file contains the experiment design for the stress condition developed in E-Prime package E-Studio 2.0. To understand the trial procedure, please see the experiment design as mentioned in Section 2.4.6.

2.8 RELEVANT PAPERS

This section provides a list of some of the papers that have utilized the data acquired from the experiment described in this chapter. The following papers should be cited when using the experiment design or the data provided in this chapter.

1. Subhani R, Malik AS, Kamel N, Saad N, Nandagopal D. "Experimental evidence for the effects of the Demand-Control model on the cognitive arousal: An EEG based study," in *Engineering in Medicine and Biology Society (EMBC), 2015 37th Annual International Conference of the IEEE*, 2015, pp. 6038–6041.
2. Subhani R, Likun X, Malik AS, Othman Z. "Quantification of physiological disparities and task performance in stress and control conditions," in *Engineering in Medicine and Biology Society (EMBC), 2013 35th Annual International Conference of the IEEE*, 2013, pp. 2060–2063.

ACKNOWLEDGMENTS

This chapter provides the details of the experiment design available in the papers mentioned in Section 2.8 and in the MS thesis of Mr. Ahmad Rauf Subhani, which is available at Universiti Teknologi PETRONAS.

REFERENCES

1. Subhani AR, Xia L, Malik AS, Othman Z. Quantification of physiological disparities and task performance in stress and control conditions. *Paper presented at: 2013 35th Annual International Conference of the IEEE Engineering in Medicine and Biology Society (EMBC)*, July 3–7, 2013.
2. Amin HU, Malik AS, Ahmad RF, et al. Feature extraction and classification for EEG signals using wavelet transform and machine learning techniques. *Australas Phys Eng Sci Med*. 2015;38(1):139–149.
3. Amin HU, Malik AS, Kamel N, Hussain M. A novel approach based on data redundancy for feature extraction of EEG signals. *Brain Topogr*. 2016;29(2):207–217.
4. Amin HU, Malik AS, Badruddin N, Kamel N, Hussain M. Effects of stereoscopic 3D display technology on event-related potentials (ERPs). *Paper presented at: Neural Engineering (NER), 2015 7th International IEEE/EMBS Conference*, April 22–24, 2015.
5. Eskelinen L, Toikkanen J, Tuomi K, Mauno I, Nygård C-H, Ilmarinen J. Symptoms of mental and physical stress in different categories of municipal work. *Scand J Work Environ Health*. 1991:82–86.
6. Deimling GT, Bass DM. Symptoms of mental impairment among elderly adults and their effects on family caregivers. *J Gerontol*. 1986;41(6):778–784.
7. De Kloet ER, Oitzl MS, Joëls M. Stress and cognition: are corticosteroids good or bad guys? *Trends Neurosci*. 1999;22(10):422–426.
8. Sapolsky RM. Stress hormones: good and bad. *Neurobiol Dis*. 2000;7(5):540–542.
9. Pressman SD, Cohen S. Does positive affect influence health? *Psychol Bull*. 2005;131(6):925.

10. The Impact of Stress. 2011; http://www.apa.org/news/press/releases/stress/2011/impact.aspx. Accessed August 29, 2016.
11. Work related stress, anxiety and depression statistics in Great Britain 2014/15. 2015; http://www.hse.gov.uk/statistics/causdis/stress/. Accessed August 29, 2016.
12. Cohen S. Perceived stress in a probability sample of the United States; 1988.
13. Cohen S, Kamarck T, Mermelstein R. A global measure of perceived stress. *J Health Soc Behav*. 1983:385–396.
14. Ursin H, Eriksen HR. The cognitive activation theory of stress. *Psychoneuroendocrinology*. 2004;29(5):567–592.
15. Lederbogen F, Kirsch P, Haddad L, et al. City living and urban upbringing affect neural social stress processing in humans. *Nature*. 2011;474(7352):498–501.
16. Dedovic K, Renwick R, Mahani NK, Engert V, Lupien SJ, Pruessner JC. The Montreal imaging stress task: using functional imaging to investigate the effects of perceiving and processing psychosocial stress in the human brain. *J Psychiatry Neurosci*. 2005;30(5):319–325.
17. Setz C, Arnrich B, Schumm J, La Marca R, Tröster G, Ehlert U. Discriminating stress from cognitive load using a wearable EDA device. *IEEE Trans Inf Technol Biomed*. 2010;14(2):410–417.
18. Williams LJ, Krishnan A, Abdi H. *Companion for Experimental Design and Analysis for Psychology*. New York: Oxford University Press; 2009.
19. Kirschbaum C, Pirke KM, Hellhammer DH. The "Trier social stress test"—A tool for investigating psychobiological stress responses in a laboratory setting. *Neuropsychobiology*. 1993;28(1–2):76–81.
20. Pruessner JC, Hellhammer DH, Kirschbaum C. Low self-esteem, induced failure and the adrenocortical stress response. *Pers Individ Dif*. 1999;27(3):477–489.

CHAPTER 3

Major Depressive Disorder

Contents

3.1 INTRODUCTION

Treatment management for major depressive disorder (MDD) has been challenging and has been associated with low treatment efficacy. Antidepressants, selective serotonin reuptake inhibitors (SSRIs), are considered to be the first line of treatment for MDD. There are more than 20 different medicines for SSRIs that are available commercially. However, the challenge lies in the appropriate selection of an antidepressant for the MDD patient. According to the existing clinical practice, the selection is based on subjective assessment with less scientific evidence. There is no guarantee that the selected antidepressant would work for the patient. To improve upon this situation, we have proposed utilization of electroencephalographic (EEG) data from the patients at baseline. EEG has the capability to capture the changes occurring inside the brain due to

Designing EEG Experiments for Studying the Brain.
DOI: http://dx.doi.org/10.1016/B978-0-12-811140-6.00003-5
© 2017 Elsevier Inc.
All rights reserved.
47

depression and anxiety.[1] However, extracting useful information from raw EEG requires computational techniques to analyze and infer such changes.[2,3] As a result, the evidence about the treatment outcome from a certain antidepressant such as SSRIs is generated, which is helpful for the psychiatrist as a second opinion. Selection of appropriate antidepressants at pretreatment stage would sufficiently reduce the multiple trials and would improve the treatment efficacy associated with MDD. In this chapter, details about this project are provided, such as sample size calculation, details about experiment design, data acquisition, and study participants.

3.2 IMPORTANCE OF STUDYING MDD

MDD or clinical depression is a common and serious mood disorder. It is a medical condition that includes abnormalities of mood, sleep, appetite, cognition, and psychomotor activity. It is among the most burdensome diseases worldwide, and as such has considerable adverse effects on the daily lives of individuals, increasing the cost of healthcare and reducing the efficiency of the workforce. In the age range of 15–44 years, it is a top cause of functional disability and the estimated economic burden of depression was $83.1 billion (including $26.1 billion medical costs, $5.54 billion suicide-related mortality costs, and $51.5 billion indirect workplace costs) in 2000 in the United States.[4,5] The high medical costs arise due to treatment nonresponse and because initial treatment is not effective for recovery[6]; e.g, one study reported a response rate of 47% with initial treatment.[7]

The reported treatment of MDD patients is through two methods: psychotherapy and pharmacotherapy. Psychotherapy includes cognitive behavioral therapy (CBT) and interpersonal therapy (IPT). CBT deals with the cognition of the patients as depression is considered to be maintained by distorted and biased cognition that affects the patient's view. CBT links a collaborative working relationship between the clinicians and the patients. It has been shown that CBT is superior to placebo and no treatment conditions.[8–11] However, the relative efficacy of CBT in comparison with psychotropic medications is questionable when dealing with severe depression patients.[12] In addition, for patients with many complex mental issues such as personality and emotional issues, there is no scope within CBT for personal exploration and assessment of emotion. IPT differs from CBT in that IPT addresses interpersonal relationships to better the patient's communications skills and self-concept.[13] It has been shown that IPT is as effective as CBT in general.[14,15] However, IPT may be less effective than CBT for MDD patients with personality disorders.[16]

The pharmacotherapy for treatment of MDD patients includes tricyclic antidepressants (TCAs), monoamine oxidase inhibitors (MAOIs), and SSRIs. TCAs are an older generation of antidepressants and are well studied and shown to be effective in up to 50–75% of patients.[16] However, there are many issues with TCAs. For example, overdose of these drugs can cause death, and side effects (blurred vision, dry mouth, drowsiness, weight gain, difficulty urinating, sexual dysfunction, etc.) are difficult to handle, resulting in 30–40% of patients terminating their use of these drugs. The MAOIs have been shown to be as effective for MDD patients as the TCAs and also effective for some nonrespondent patients.[17,18] Besides, these drugs also have many limitations, resulting in infrequent use. An issue with MAOIs is that there is potential interaction with other substances that can cause severe consequences, i.e., foods containing tyramine must be avoided during the use of these drugs. In addition, similar to TCAs, an overdose of these drugs can be severe. The side effects of MAOIs include weight gain, sedation, and orthostatic hypotension. Now the first line of MDD treatment is the new class of antidepressant called SSRIs. It has been shown that this new class of antidepressant is more effective than other antidepressants.[19–21] The side effects of SSRIs as compared to TCAs and other antidepressants are minor and transient. The common side effects of SSRIs are headaches, decrease in appetite and sexual desires, and nausea. In addition, an overdose of SSRIs is safe but they are relatively expensive compared to TCAs. However, some studies reported similar compliance rates for SSRIs with other antidepressants.[22]

Despite all these available medications for MDD treatment, there is an issue for clinicians as well as for the patients. Since each pharmacotherapy class contains multiple antidepressants, e.g., the SSRIs include more than 20 antidepressants, the challenge is how to select a suitable antidepressant for a certain MDD patient. In the present clinical practice, many clinicians use a trial-and-error approach while recommending antidepressants to MDD patients; selection of antidepressants is also based on subjective assessment, which is a costly and inefficient way of treatment. Furthermore, the initial treatment or assessment of antidepressant efficacy needs 2–4 weeks. In case the antidepressant is not effective, the clinicians require changing the antidepressant and recommending a new one, which will also need around 2–4 weeks of time. This practice is time consuming, costly, and may increase the severity of depression in a particular patient due to prolonged treatment duration. This happens because of the absence of scientific evidence in the initial treatment and the patient's diagnosis. To cope with such practices, the antidepressants require a scientific prediction for their efficacy about the patient's treatment. Hence, quantitative assessment based on neuroimaging techniques such as EEG will support the clinicians in assessing the effectiveness of a particular antidepressant for a particular MDD patient.[23,24]

3.3 PROBLEM STATEMENT

Generally, the treatment management for MDD has been largely based on subjective assessments. Further, there are more than 20 different antidepressants commercially available under the category of SSRIs. However, for a particular patient, suitable selection of an antidepressant is challenging and may end up as a trial-and-error approach. Studies involving prediction of treatment efficacy for MDD have shown promising results. However, there is still a need to address this issue and improve the prediction of treatment efficacy. The issues in the existing prediction studies include low efficiencies and differences in the methodological procedures adopted. There is a clear need for objective measures that can predict treatment efficacies for MDD.

3.4 SOFTWARE/HARDWARE

In this study, EEG data was recorded using a 24-channel BrainMaster Discovery EEG with the manufacturer's acquisition software. Data was acquired using the DC amplifier with 19-channel EEG sensor cap. The Discovery software was linked with E-Prime software for controlling the time-locked visual stimuli tasks such as the oddball task. After the data acquisition, the raw EEG signals were preprocessed using BESA research v.6.0 software. The clean EEG signals were processed in MATLAB for advanced analysis and feature extraction. The details of this hardware and software are provided below.

BrainMaster DC Amplifier: BrainMaster Discovery amplifier (Fig. 3.1) is designed to provide EEG signals from DC (0 Hz) to 80 Hz with 24-bit accuracy. The specifications of the amplifier are described as follows:

- *Channels*: 24 (19 EEG channels used based on 10–20 electrode placement)
- A/D accuracy: 24 bits; resolution 0.01 microvolts EEG, 0.4 microvolts DC

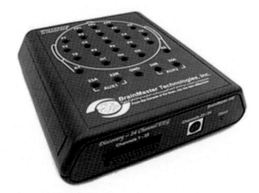

Figure 3.1 BrainMaster Discovery amplifier.

- Amplifier bandwidth: 0.000–100 Hz
- EEG channel bandwidth: 0.43–80 Hz
- DC offset signal bandwidth: 0.000–2 Hz
- Input noise <1.0 microvolt RMS (0.43–60 Hz)
- Sampling rate: 512 samples/second
- Data rate to PC: 256 samples/second
- Connection to PC: USB, optically and magnetically isolated
- Software supported (live acquisition): BrainMaster Discovery, NeuroGuide Live
- Software supported (analysis via EDF files): NeuroGuide, SKIL, WinEEG, Persyst, EDF Browser, other

BrainMaster Discovery acquisition software: BrainMaster Discovery software is designed for Windows XP, Vista, Win 7, and Win 8. This software is not open source and requires a license to operate it. The user interface of the Discovery software is shown in Fig. 3.2.

E-Prime: E-Prime software is designed for stimulus presentation during the experiment and is synchronized with the corresponding EEG amplifier (http://www.pstnet.com). Time-locked evoked potentials can be recorded using BrainMaster Discovery software along with the E-Prime software. The timing information can be sent to the Discovery software via a cable (381-017) that connects the PC parallel port to channels 23 and 24 of the Discovery data. Stim pulses will appear in one or both of these channels.

BESA Research 6.0: Brain Electrical Source Analysis (BESA) software was mainly developed for source analysis and dipole localization in EEG and magnetoencephalogram (MEG) signals. However, it has implemented state-of-the-art artifact removal methods such as ICA-based automatic

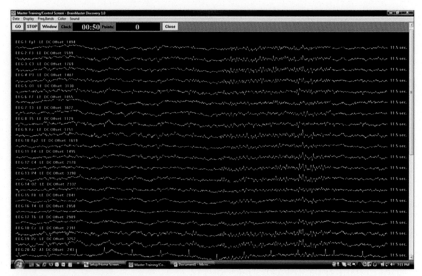

Figure 3.2 User interface of BrainMaster Discovery acquisition software.

cleaning and Berg's method of electrooculogram (EOG) artifact removal. It allows rereferencing the raw data and exporting clean EEG data in many file formats such as .edf and .mat. Its user-friendly interface allows researchers to apply filters on raw EEG, remove EOG artifacts, ECG artifacts, line noise, and other high-frequency artifacts such as muscle artifacts.

MATLAB: MATLAB is a high-performance programming language for technical computing and coding for engineering problems. It provides an integrative environment for use by engineers and scientists worldwide. The easy-to-use programming environment of MATLAB provides fast solutions to complex mathematical problems. The well-known disciplines of MATLAB programming are signal and image processing, communications and control systems, computational neuroscience and GUI (graphical user interface) programming, pattern recognition and machine learning. For beginners in neuroscience, the book *MATLAB for Neuroscientists* by Pascal Wallisch and colleagues can be consulted.

3.5 EXPERIMENT DESIGN AND PROTOCOL

3.5.1 Target Population

The target population for this study were MDD patients in Malaysia. However, the selection of the potential participants from the MDD patients was based on the inclusion criteria as defined in the next subsection.

3.5.2 Inclusion Criteria

The following inclusion criteria were defined for the participant to be involved in the experiment:

1. Patients must sign written informed consent
2. Patients must be within the age limit (18–65 years)
3. Patients with diagnosed MDD (DSM-IV)
   a. Newly diagnosed (new cases)
   b. Newly started (old cases)
      i. Restarted on antidepressant (one week washout)
      ii. Switched to new antidepressant

3.5.3 Exclusion Criteria

Patients were excluded in the study based on the following exclusion criteria:

1. Patients having psychotic, cognitive disorder
2. Patients with any other drug abuse
3. Pregnant patients
4. Patients with epilepsy

3.5.4 Clinical Questionnaires

The clinical datasets include assessment scores based on clinically relevant questionnaires such as the Hospital Anxiety and Depression Scale (HADS) and the Beck Depression Inventory II (BDI-II). For this study, the questionnaires were Malay (national language in Malaysia) translated versions. The Malay versions of HADS[25] and BDI-II[26] are standard clinically proven questionnaires to rate MDD severity. Furthermore, the questionnaires were self-administered. However, to improve the quality and to maintain the accuracy of the process, the questionnaires were administered under the supervision of an experienced nursing staff.

3.5.5 Sample Size Computation

In this study, a group of 33 MDD patients were recruited based on the given formula.[27,28]

$$n = \frac{P(1 - P) \cdot (Z_{1-\alpha/2})^2}{e^2}$$

where P is the expected proportion (e.g., expected diagnostic sensitivity); e is the error limit, which is one half the desired width of the confidence interval; and $Z_{1-\alpha/2}$ is the standard normal Z value corresponding to a cumulative probability of $1- \alpha/2$. The investigator must specify the best guess for the proportion that is expected to be found after performing the study.[2] The recommended threshold for the statistical parameters used in the computation of the sample size was defined as follows:

- significance $\alpha = 0.05$ (alpha)
- power of test $= 80\%, \beta = 0.2$ (Beta)
- expected diagnostic accuracy[29] $P = 90.5\%$
- expected error $e = 10\%$

Therefore, for statistical parameters $P = 0.905$, $\alpha = 0.05$, $e = 0.10$, $Z_{1-\alpha/2} = 1.96$, the sample size is calculated as follows:

$$n = \frac{(0.905)(0.095)(1.96)^2}{(0.10)^2} = 33$$

3.5.6 Participant Recruitment

In this study, 33 MDD outpatients (16 males and 17 females, mean age $= 40.33 \pm 12.861$) were recruited from the psychiatry clinic at Hospital Universiti Sains Malaysia (HUSM) with signed consent forms. The patients met the internationally recognized diagnostic criteria for depression, as defined in the *Diagnostic and Statistical Manual* IV (DSM-IV).[30] In addition, a second group including 19 age-matched normal controls (8 males and 10 females, mean age $= 38.277 \pm 15.64$) was also recruited. The normal controls were examined medically and were found to be without any psychiatric conditions. The participants from both groups were briefed about the experiment design before its commencement. For MDD patients, after completing 2 weeks of washout time period, the first session of EEG data acquisition was carried out. After the first EEG session, the patients started taking the antidepressants under the general category of SSRIs (see Table 3.1).

3.5.7 Ethics Approval

The experimental design protocol for this study was approved by the Research Ethics Committee of the Hospital Universiti Sains Malaysia (HUSM), Kelantan, Malaysia (FWA Reg. No. 00007718; IRB Reg. No. 00004494). The Subject Information and Consent Form is provided in Appendix 2C.

Table 3.1 Available clinical characteristics of SSRI responders and nonresponders who participated in the study

Information	R	NR	Total	p values
Age (years)	40.733 (±13.0245)	41.176 (±12.47)	40.33 (±12.861)	0.9224
Gender (female/male)	8/7	9/8	17/16	0.9896
Pretreatment BDI	18.444 (±7.384)	22.8235 (±12.476)	20.633 (±8.582)	0.2521
Pretreatment HADS	11 (±1.581)	10.454 (±3.297)	10.727 (±2.439)	0.7336
SSRI treatment[a]	E:9,F:2,S:4,Fl:1	E:4,F:7,S:4,Fl:2	E:13,F:9,S:8,Fl:3	

Mean (±standard deviation) are shown for the relevant variables
[a]SSRI medication administered: *E*, Escitalopram; *F*, Fluvoxamine; *S*, Sertraline; *Fl*, Fluxetine

3.6 EXPERIMENTAL TASKS AND PROCEDURE

3.6.1 Procedure/Methodology

An interventional study with dependent sample of MDD patients ($n = 33$) was carried out. The duration of the study was 4 weeks. MDD patients meeting exclusion/inclusion criteria were selected and medicated with an antidepressant. The patients were recruited from the psychiatry department of HUSM. Recruitment procedure was based on their willingness and was carried out by the researcher. Patients were given a demonstration about the experiment and research information (see Appendix 14) and an informed consent was given (see Appendix 2C). After signing the consent form, a data collection form was filled out based on their demographic information.

Fig. 3.3 explains the data collection scheme. Two types of data collection were involved: electrophysiological (EEG) data and clinical assessments using the HADS (Appendix 3A) and BDI-II (Appendix 3B) questionnaires. For EEG data, a wearable 24-channel cap and equipment were used. A total of five recording sessions of both types of recordings were performed. The first recording session, also known as the baseline, was carried out when the patients were unmedicated for at least the past two weeks. The second recording session was done one week after the start of medication. EEG recordings and clinical assessments were carried out after each week for the remaining sessions.

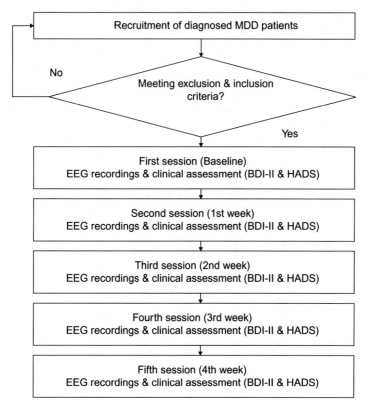

Figure 3.3 Data collection scheme.

EEG data collection consisted of the four steps seen in Fig. 3.4. A total of 40 minutes was required.

Step 1 was to set up the experiment using a 24–channel wearable cap. The suitable cap was selected by measuring patients' head size using a head measuring tape. Proper setting up of the cap was important for data quality. This process took about 20 minutes.

Step 2 is eyes closed (EC) session: patients were required to sit on a chair with eyes closed and not fall asleep. This took about 5 minutes.

Step 3 was the eyes–open (EO) session: patients were required to look at a fixation point ("+") on a computer screen in front of them with minimal eye movements or blinking. This required nearly 5 minutes.

Step 4 was a visual three-stimulus oddball task: patients were exposed to a random sequence of shapes on a computer screen. Only one shape was displayed at a time. There were a total of three shapes (Fig. 3.5): target

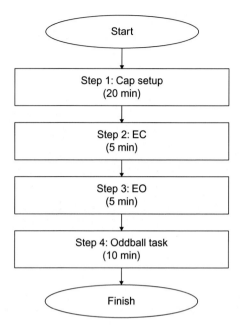

Figure 3.4 EEG data collection.

Category	Stimulus		Component
Target (0.12)	5.0 cm	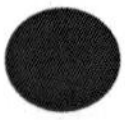 ⬤	P3b (P300)
Distracter (0.12)	18.0 cm	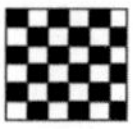 ▦	P3a
Standard (0.76)	4.5 cm	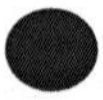 ⬤	N1, P2, N2 (Sensory potentials)

Category = P3a/P3b stimulus type (probability). Stimulus = physical characteristics and width. Component = potentials produced for specific conditions. Blue circles were presented on light gray background and the checkerboard was composed of black and white checks approximately 1 cm square.

Figure 3.5 Visual three-stimulus oddball task.[31]

(a blue circle) with 5.0 cm size; standard (a blue circle) with 4.5 cm size; and distractor (a checker board) with 18.0 cm size.

Patients must respond to the target shape by pressing the SPACE key on the keyboard, but no action must be taken in response to other shapes. This process took about 10 minutes.

3.7 DATA DESCRIPTION

There is no behavioral data collected during the EEG recording. However, the clinical assessments involved the usage of questionnaires such as BDI-II and HADS.

The EEG data was recorded in resting state conditions and while performing the oddball task (event-related potentials—ERP) five times over the period of four weeks. The oddball data consisted of 314 standard trials, 45 target trials, and 41 distractor trials. The EEG raw data were saved in .edf file format. According to the experimental protocol, the intervention duration was four weeks and the subjects were observed five times, i.e., at week0, week1, week2, week3, and week4. The "week0" data is recorded at start of the intervention and considered as baseline data; while week1 to week4 data were recorded exactly after each week time. The EEG clean data was saved in .mat format. Each week's data consisted of three files. The details of these files are provided in Table 3.2. To access these files, please go to the directory BookData\Chap03 in the data files accompanying this book. It is to be noted that the raw and clean data for one subject are provided in separate directories. For the complete dataset of 33 participants, please contact the authors of this book at brainexpbook@gmail.com.

3.8 RELEVANT PAPERS

This section provides a list of some of the papers that have utilized the data acquired from the experiment described in this chapter. The following papers should be cited when using the experiment design or the data provided with this chapter.

1. Mumtaz W, Malik AS, Yasin MAM, Xia L. Review on EEG and ERP predictive biomarkers for major depressive disorder. *Biomed Signal Process Control* 2015;22:85–98.
2. Mumtaz W, Malik AS, Ali SSA, Yasin MAM, Amin HU. Detrended fluctuation analysis for major depressive disorder. In: *Engineering in Medicine and Biology Society (EMBC), 2015 37th Annual International Conference of the IEEE*; 2015, pp. 4162–4165.

ACKNOWLEDGMENTS

This chapter provides the details of the experiment design available in the papers mentioned in Section 3.8 and in the PhD thesis of Wajid Mumtaz, which is available at Universiti Teknologi PETRONAS.

Table 3.2 Description of EEG data files and E-Prime file

S. No.	File name	Description
01	EC.edf	Resting state EEG recording at eyes-closed condition (provided for 5 weeks)
02	EO.edf	Resting state EEG recording at eyes-open condition (provided for 5 weeks)
03	ERP.edf	EEG data recorded during performing oddball task (provided for 5 weeks). The ERP signals can be extracted by detecting the visual stimulus events using channels 23 or 24 in discovery data.
04	Event File.xlsx	This event file contains the events information of the oddball task (ERP). This file can be accessed from BookData\Chap03\EEG Data\EEG Raw Data. The event file contains time stamps of ERP data recorded in five different times, i.e., week0, week1 … week4. There are 400 events and three categories of stimuli (shape). The time stamps of each recording are listed in the event file as a column.
05	Oddball Task	This experiment is designed in E-Prime software, which can be accessed from BookData\Chap03\Experiment Design\Oddball Task. The task contains three visual stimuli as shown in Fig. 3.5. The experiment can only be opened in E-Prime software.

REFERENCES

1. Cavanagh J, Geisler MW. Mood effects on the ERP processing of emotional intensity in faces: a P3 investigation with depressed students. *Int J Psychophysiol.* 2006;60(1):27–33.
2. Amin HU, Malik AS, Kamel N, Hussain M. A novel approach based on data redundancy for feature extraction of EEG signals. *Brain Topogr.* 2016;29(2):207–217.
3. Amin HU, Malik AS, Ahmad RF, et al. Feature extraction and classification for EEG signals using wavelet transform and machine learning techniques. *Australas Phys Eng Sci Med.* 2015;38(1):139–149.
4. Merikangas KR, Ames M, Cui L, et al. The impact of comorbidity of mental and physical conditions on role disability in the US adult household population. *Arch Gen Psychiatry.* 2007;64(10):1180–1188.
5. Greenberg PE, Kessler RC, Birnbaum HG, et al. The economic burden of depression in the United States: how did it change between 1990 and 2000? *J Clin Psychiatry.* 2003;64(12):1465–1475.
6. Simon GE, Khandker RK, Ichikawa L, Operskalski BH. Recovery from depression predicts lower health services costs. *J Clin Psychiatry.* 2006;67(8):1226–1231.
7. Trivedi MH, Rush AJ, Wisniewski SR, et al. Evaluation of outcomes with citalopram for depression using measurement-based care in STAR★D: implications for clinical practice. *Am J Psychiatry.* 2006;163(1):28–40.
8. Dobson KS. A meta-analysis of the efficacy of cognitive therapy for depression. *J Consult Clin Psychol.* 1989;57(3):414.

9. Gaffan E, Tsaousis J, Kemp-Wheeler S. Researcher allegiance and meta-analysis: the case of cognitive therapy for depression. *J Consult Clin Psychol*. 1995;63(6):966.

10. Blackburn I, Moore R. Controlled acute and follow-up trial of cognitive therapy and pharmacotherapy in out-patients with recurrent depression. *Br J Psychiatry*. 1997;171(4):328–334.

11. Gloaguen V, Cottraux J, Cucherat M, Blackburn I-M. A meta-analysis of the effects of cognitive therapy in depressed patients. *J Affect Disord*. 1998;49(1):59–72.

12. Hamilton KE, Dobson KS. Cognitive therapy of depression: pretreatment patient predictors of outcome. *Clin Psychol Rev*. 2002;22(6):875–893.

13. Weissman MM, Markowitz JC. *Interpersonal Psychotherapy of Depression*. Jason Aronson, Incorporated; 1994.

14. Collins JF, Elkin I, Sotsky SM, Docherty JP. Personality disorders and treatment outcome in the NIMH Treatment of Depression Collaborative Research Program. *Am J Psychiatry*. 1990;147:711–718.

15. Clark DM, Salkovskis PM, Hackmann A, Middleton H, Anastasiades P, Gelder M. A comparison of cognitive therapy, applied relaxation and imipramine in the treatment of panic disorder. *Br J Psychiatry*. 1994;164(6):759–769.

16. Hardy GE, Barkham M, Shapiro DA, Reynolds S, Rees A, Stiles WB. Credibility and outcome of cognitive—behavioural and psychodynamic—interpersonal psychotherapy. *Br J Clin Psychol*. 1995;34(4):555–569.

17. Thase ME, Greenhouse JB, Frank E, et al. Treatment of major depression with psychotherapy or psychotherapy-pharmacotherapy combinations. *Arch Gen Psychiatry*. 1997;54(11):1009–1015.

18. Zisook S, Braff DL, Click MA. Monoamine oxidase inhibitors in the treatment of atypical depression. *J Clin Psychopharmacol*. 1985;5(3):131 137.

19. Anderson I, Tomenson B. Treatment discontinuation with selective serotonin reuptake inhibitors compared with tricyclic antidepressants: a meta-analysis. *BMJ*. 1995;310(6992):1433–1438.

20. Anderson IM. Selective serotonin reuptake inhibitors versus tricyclic antidepressants: a meta-analysis of efficacy and tolerability. *J Affect Disord*. 2000;58(1):19–36.

21. MacGillivray S, Arroll B, Hatcher S, et al. Efficacy and tolerability of selective serotonin reuptake inhibitors compared with tricyclic antidepressants in depression treated in primary care: systematic review and meta-analysis. *BMJ*. 2003;326(7397):1014.

22. Trindade E, Menon D, Topfer L-A, Coloma C. Adverse effects associated with selective serotonin reuptake inhibitors and tricyclic antidepressants: a meta-analysis. *Can Med Assoc J*. 1998;159(10):1245–1252.

23. Mumtaz W, Malik AS, Yasin MAM, Xia L. Review on EEG and ERP predictive biomarkers for major depressive disorder. *Biomed Signal Process Control*. 2015;22:85–98.

24. Mumtaz W, Xia L, Ali SSA, Yasin MAM, Hussain M, Malik AS. Electroencephalogram (EEG)-based computer-aided technique to diagnose major depressive disorder (MDD). *Biomed Signal Process Control*. 2017;31:108–115.

25. Yusoff N, Low WY, Yip C-H. Psychometric properties of the Malay Version of the hospital anxiety and depression scale: a study of husbands of breast cancer patients in Kuala Lumpur, Malaysia. *Asian Pac J Cancer Prevent*. 2011;12(4):915–917.

26. Mahmud WMRW, Awang A, Herman I, Mohamed MN. Analysis of the psychometric properties of the Malay version of Beck Depression Inventory II (BDI-II) among postpartum women in Kedah, north west of peninsular Malaysia. *Malays J Med Sci MJMS*. 2004;11(2):19.

27. Fosgate GT. Practical sample size calculation for surveillance and diagnostic investigations. *J Vet Diagn Investig*. 2009;21:3–14.

28. Zhou XH, Obuchowski NA, McClish DK. Statistical Methods in Diagnostic Medicine. In: Statistics Wsipa, ed: Wiley series in probability and statistics; 2002.

29. Khodayari-Rostamabad A, Hasey GM, MacCrimmon DJ, Reilly JP, Bruin Hd. A pilot study to determine whether machine learning methodologies using pre-treatment electroencephalography can predict the symptomatic response to clozapine therapy. *Clin Neurophysiol.* 2010;121:1998–2006.
30. Association AP. Diagnostic and statistical manual of mental disorders: DSM-IV-TR®. American Psychiatric Pub; 2000.
31. Polich J, Criado JR. Neuropsychology and neuropharmacology of P3a and P3b. *Int J Psychophysiol.* 2006;60:172–185.

CHAPTER 4

Epileptic Seizures

Contents

4.1 INTRODUCTION

Epilepsy is a chronic brain disorder that involves recurrent seizure activity. Clinically, the epileptic seizure activity can be defined as "intermittent paroxysmal, stereotyped disturbance of consciousness, behavior, emotion, motor function, perception, or sensation, which may occur singly or in combination and is thought to be the result of abnormal cortical neuronal discharges."[1] However, seizures originating from certain brain regions and the affected range may differentiate the type of seizure activity. The origination and development of epilepsy may cause abnormalities in synaptic transmission and neuronal excitability.[1]

According to the World Health Organization (WHO), it is reported that epileptic disorder is among the most primary diseases of the brain. The statistics show that there are more than 50 million in the world people suffering from epileptic disorder and most of the affected people are living in the developing countries (around 80%), where the health facilities are not satisfactory. The treatment can be in the form of medicines or the removal of brain epileptogenic tissues in severe cases; however, the surgery may result in disturbance of the routine functions of the human body due to removal of brain tissues.[2,3] A general scenario of visualization of epilepsy attack is shown in Fig. 4.1.

Designing EEG Experiments for Studying the Brain.
DOI: http://dx.doi.org/10.1016/B978-0-12-811140-6.00004-7
© 2017 Elsevier Inc.
All rights reserved.

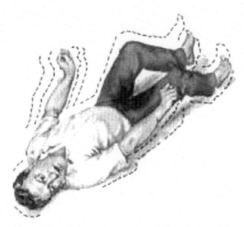

Figure 4.1 A general scenario of epileptic seizure attack.[4]

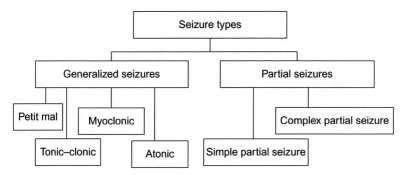

Figure 4.2 Epileptic seizure categories.

4.1.1 Classification of Epileptic Seizures

The epileptic seizure can be classified into two main categories, i.e., generalized seizures and partial seizures. The difference between these seizures is how and where they start in the brain (see Fig. 4.2). Generalized seizures involve both hemispheres and begin with a widespread electrical discharge at once. However, partial seizures begin with limited area of the brain and may spread to other brain regions. Generalized seizures have further categories such as petit mal, tonic–clonic, myoclonic, and atonic seizures. Partial seizures have also two further categories, i.e., simple partial and complex partial seizures.[1]

4.1.1.1 Generalized Seizures

- Petit mal: This type of seizure is also known as an absence seizure. The symptom of absence seizure is a brief loss of consciousness. Patients suffering from absence seizures may not be aware that they are having seizures. It may occur several times a day and have an abrupt start and end. Children suffering from absence seizures will stare blankly during seizure activity. The duration of unconsciousness is around a few seconds.[1]

- Tonic–clonic: Tonic–clonic or grand mal seizures cause convulsions, muscle rigidity, and unconsciousness. They are differentiated by stiffening of muscles. A patient may lose consciousness for a small duration of time during the tonic phase. Further, the body of the patient starts shaking and stretching and causes muscular contractions.[1]
- Myoclonic: This kind of seizure causes small jerks on both sides of the body.[1] The patients may feel the jerks as brief electrical shocks; if violent, it may result in throwing objects involuntarily.
- Atonic: This consists of sudden lack of muscle control especially in the arms and legs and the duration is usually around 15 seconds.[1]

4.1.1.2 Partial Seizures

- Simple partial seizures: This kind of seizure occurs in just one area. The symptoms of this seizure are muscle contractions, visual disturbances, and blackouts, but for very brief duration, like a minute or less than a minute. The patients may feel fearful and anxious during partial seizures.[1]
- Complex partial seizures: In complex partial seizures, the patients may suffer from loss of consciousness and the duration of seizures may be around a minute or two. The patients may feel uneasiness or nausea before the seizure activity.[1]

4.2 IMPORTANCE OF STUDYING EPILEPSY

There is a rich literature available on epilepsy detection system–based electroencephalography (EEG) signals and computational techniques. The various epileptic seizure detection techniques have been developed based on EEG signals using linear and nonlinear methods.[5,6] These techniques mainly include feature extraction methods along with machine-learning algorithms to discriminate between seizure, seizure-free, and normal EEG patterns. These methods include frequency domain analysis (e.g., subbands analysis), entropy analysis, wavelet analysis, largest Lyapunov exponent, correlation dimension, fractal dimension, Hurst exponent, and higher-order cumulants.[6,7] Machine-learning algorithms used in these techniques include artificial neural network (ANN), k-nearest neighbor (k-NN), support vector machine (SVM), naïve Bayes classifier, the Gaussian mixture model (GMM), the fuzzy classifier, and the decision tree.

Time and frequency domain techniques are normally used for feature extraction from EEG signals; extracted features are further used as inputs to the classifiers.[8] In addition to frequency domain features, researchers have commonly used discrete wavelet transform (DWT) to analyze EEG signals. DWT decomposes EEG signals into time–frequency representations. Gotman et al.[9] initially proposed an automated seizure prediction technique that was widely employed. After EEG signal decomposition, features such as peak amplitude, time-duration, sharpness, and slope were used to detect epileptic seizure activity. Khan et al. used the DWT to decompose EEG signals into subbands from which features including energy and coefficient variation were computed and used to detect seizure activity. Adeli et al.[10,11] used the wavelet transform to analyze and characterize the epileptic discharge as a 3 Hz spike. Using wavelet decomposition, transient features were accurately computed and localized in time and frequency domains. Subasi et al.[12] proposed a method based on wavelet transform and ANNs to classify EEG seizure signals. Subasi's team[13] later improved their method by using dynamic fuzzy neural networks. Guo et al.[14] employed automatic feature extraction based on genetic programming (GP) to classify epileptic seizure signals. In 2014, Kumar et al.[15] classified EEG signals based on features computed via fuzzy approximate entropy (fApEn) and DWT. Senhadji et al.[8] used wavelet transform for time-duration analysis and a time–frequency approach to analyze the spectral content of EEG signals as a function of time. The same authors utilized both approaches to detect interictal spikes and to determine the ictal period. Tzallas et al.[16] employed time–frequency analysis using many time–frequency distributions including short-time Fourier transform (STFT) with four different classification algorithms for epileptic seizure detection. However, ANNs achieved high classification results. Das et al.[17] proposed a seizure detection method using symmetric normal inverse Gaussian parameters of subbands of EEG computed in dual-tree complex wavelet transformation. SVM with radial-basis function (RBF) kernel was used for classification of seizure from nonseizure EEG patterns. Besides, chaotic feature extraction techniques have been used for epileptic seizure detection, such as largest Lyapunov exponent, Hurst exponent, and fractal dimension, reported by Hosseini et al.[18,19] The combination of chaotic features and adaptive neuro fuzzy inference system classifier achieved 98.6% accuracy for classification of normal from interictal EEG patterns and 98.1% accuracy for separating ictal from normal signals. Chen et al.[20] proposed a method to reduce the computational load for the classical wavelet transform. Further, ANNs and logistic regression were used to classify epileptic seizure activity. Xie et al.[21] developed a sparse functional linear model based on wavelets to represent EEG signals using wavelet variance to capture discriminative components in EEG signals. Acharya et al.[22] decomposed EEG signals into wavelet coefficients by using wavelet packet decomposition. They removed eigenvalues from these coefficients with the help of principal component analysis (PCA). ANOVA of eigenvalues then identified those of significance. Further classifiers were trained using 10-fold cross-validation techniques. The GMM classifier was also used to obtain high classification accuracy for epileptic signals. Wang et al.[23] used wavelet packet entropy for feature extractions that achieved a hierarchical classification approach. Recently, Kumar et al.[15] proposed a wavelet-based fuzzy-approximate entropy (fApEn) method to SVM for classification purposes. Discrete wavelet transforms decomposed EEG signals into subfrequency bands. The fApEN of each subband was then computed to assess the chaotic behavior of EEG signals. The highest classification level achieved used SVM with the RBF kernel.

Upadhyay et al.[24] computed wavelet fractal features from wavelet coefficients of four subbands extracted using different wavelets, such as Haar, biorthogonal, Coiflets, and Daubechies, for epileptic seizure detection. Three classifiers, such as least square SVM, ANN, and random forest tree, were tested for classification of normal EEG (sets A, B) versus epileptic seizure (set E). The ANN achieved 100% accuracy with feature computed with db3 wavelet. Kumar and Kolekar[25] employed different time–frequency domain feature extraction methods such as fractal dimension, zero-crossing, subbands energy, and variance. The two classes C (interictal) versus E (ictal) were tested with SVM and reported 98% performance of seizure selection. DWT with db4 wavelet was used for feature extraction and classifying the normal and epileptic epochs using ANNs by Kulasuriya and Perera.[26] The data was decomposed up to the fifth level and 10 hidden layer neurons were used. The achieved classification accuracy was 86.67%. However, the authors employed other than Bonn datasets.

In clinical applications the diagnostic or detection system should have a high accuracy of detection. The existing literature suggests that the majority of studies were unable to achieve perfect results (100%) when attempting to detect and differentiate seizure activity from seizure-free EEG signals or seizure-free signals from normal EEG segments.

4.3 PROBLEM STATEMENT

Epilepsy is a neurological disorder involving recurrent seizure, a sudden change in behavior due to increased electrical activity inside the brain. The abnormal change in electrical activity causes unconsciousness and uncontrolled body shakes. There is no exact reason for epilepsy disorder; it may be due to inheritance, strokes, or tumors. It can severely degrade the quality of life of human beings. Around 70% of patients have intractable epilepsy. However, the seizure activity may be controlled or the frequency of occurrence can be reduced, which may help the patients to live like other normal human beings.

EEG is a brain imaging technique that has been employed for many decades to study the brain, including disorders such as epilepsy. The EEG signals help to study the neuronal abnormalities occurring due to epilepsy. The EEG recordings are composed of a huge amount of data from hours to days, which makes it quite difficult and time consuming for a medical professional to detect a seizure. In addition, EEG cannot be understood by untrained or less-experienced medical doctors. Therefore, trained professionals, neurosurgeons, and neurologists are required to interpret the EEG with seizures. In general, paramedical staff such as nurses cannot read or interpret EEG; it is difficult even for general physicians to understand EEG signals. This significantly reduces the medical professionals who have expertise of understanding EEG. Bateman[27] in 2011 surveyed that there is only one neurologist per 20,000 population in Holland and only one per 150,000 in the United Kingdom. Hence, automated seizure detection systems are supporting the doctors to examine the EEG recordings for detection of seizure activity. The automatic seizure systems are based on algorithms that are developed using computational techniques.[28,29] Medical doctors are able to automatically generate reports of epileptic seizures for a patient from long EEG recordings using seizure detection algorithms. The duration of seizure activity and the time between the occurrences of two seizures can be identified. The information on how frequently a seizure activity is occurring may be of help to prescribe a better medication or a stimulus to reduce the seizure activities.

Liu et al.[30] reported autocorrelation analysis for development of an epileptic seizure detection system independent of patient and capable of achieving 84% sensitivity. Similarly, another study conducted by Gotman[31] proposed a method for epileptic seizure detection that evaluates the EEG signal and determines the rhythmic activity. The method is capable of performing at 71% average seizure detection rate. Hassanpour[32] proposed an algorithm that is useful to determine differences between a seizure activity and a nonseizure activity using the distribution function of the singular vectors about the time–frequency distribution of EEG segments. The outcome of the algorithm is 92.5% sensitivity and was tested on 8 patients. Wilson et al.[33] proposed the "reveal algorithm," which was developed using the matching pursuit technique and achieved 76% sensitivity. Greene et al.[34] utilized both ECG and EEG signals to improve efficiency of the seizure detection method. Their algorithm is capable of accurately classifying seizure from nonseizure activity with 86.32% accuracy, 76.37% sensitivity, and 88.77% specificity.

There is a need to improve the performance of the seizure detection algorithm. Hence, it is necessary to develop a seizure event detection algorithm that could detect the seizure activity more efficiently and accurately and minimize the false detection rate of the algorithm. Furthermore, the improvement in the computational processing of the algorithm will lead to the development of real-time clinical applications for epilepsy diagnosis. In addition, epilepsy prediction research is also of paramount importance. Development of real-time methods for prediction of an epileptic seizure will drastically improve the quality of life of epileptic patients. These developments of research methods require epilepsy datasets. Fortunately, there are three epilepsy datasets available, the details of which are provided in the next section.

4.4 DETAILS OF PUBLIC EEG DATABASES

There are three well-known epilepsy datasets reported in literature and online available for research purposes. These datasets include the University of Bonn dataset, the CHB-MIT dataset, and the European Epilepsy dataset. The first two are freely available online and the last dataset needs to be paid for. The detail of these datasets is given below.

4.4.1 University of Bonn Dataset

This EEG database is publically available database provided by the University of Bonn as acquired by Andrzejak et al.[35] It comprises five datasets denoted A, B, C, D, and E. Each dataset contains 100 single-channel EEG segments with duration of 23.6 seconds totaling 4097 samples per channel; see Table 4.1 for description. Each dataset is available as a zip file containing 100 TXT files (ASCII code). Datasets were recorded with

Table 4.1 Description of Bonn datasets

Datasets	File name	Description
A	Z001.txt to Z100.txt	Sets A and B contain surface EEG recordings
B	O001.txt to O100.txt	of five healthy subjects with eyes open (EO) and eyes closed, respectively.
C	N001.txt to N100.txt	Datasets C, D, and E comprise EEG readings of five epileptic patients with sensors at various spatial locations. Dataset C contains EEG recordings from the hippocampal formation in the hemisphere opposite the epileptogenic zone.
D	F001.txt to F100.txt	Dataset D contains EEG recordings of the epileptogenic zone. Both C and D readings were recorded during seizure-free periods.
E	S001.txt to S100.txt	Set E is a collection of epileptic seizure activity recorded from the hippocampal focus.

128-channel electrodes using an average reference. Pathological activity from datasets C, D, and E and eye movement artifacts had been previously removed. For data acquisition, 12-bit analog-to-digital converters were used with a sampling frequency of 173.61 Hz. Raw EEG data had been passed from a band-pass filter ranging from 0.53 to 40 Hz with a 12 dB/oct filter roll-off.[35] Hence, EEG data is comprised of 5 (classes) × 100 (observations/class) × 4097 (23.6 seconds/observation).

4.4.2 CHB-MIT Dataset

The CHB-MIT dataset also referred to as the PhysioNet EEG dataset,[36] composed of a total of 24 pediatric patients' EEG recordings that were was acquired at Boston Children's Hospital. The patients suffered from intractable epilepsy, and the ages of the patients are between 1.5 years and 19 years. In the EEG data acquisition, the international 10–20 system of channel configuration with bipolar montage was used. The number of electrodes varies for different patients from 23 electrodes to 28 electrodes, whereas some electrodes were interchanged in some cases. The first 18 electrodes are similar for all of the patients. There are 198 total identified seizures and duration of the dataset is 916 hours. In the dataset, the epileptogenic source for the patients is not shown; though, the origins of epileptic sources were reported for each patient in another study conducted by Nasehi et al.[37] In this dataset, the shortest seizure is 6 seconds long and

Table 4.2 Description of CHB-MIT dataset

Patient no.	Gender	Age (years)	Brain region of seizure origin	Seizures counts
1	Female	11	T	7
2	Male	11	F	3
3	Female	14	T	7
4	Male	22	T, O	4
5	Female	7	F	5
6	Female	1.5	T	10
7	Female	14.5	T	3
8	Male	3.5	T	5
9	Female	10	F	4
10	Male	3	T	7
11	Female	12	F	3
12	Female	2	F	40
13	Female	3	T, O	12
14	Female	9	T	8
15	Female	16	F,T	20
16	Female	7	T	10
17	Female	12	T	3
18	Female	18	T, O	6
19	Female	19	F	3
20	Female	6	T	8
21	Female	13	T	4
22	Female	9	T, O	3
23	Female	6	F	7
24	–	–	–	16
			Total	198

F, frontal; O, occipital; T, temporal

the longest seizure duration is 752 seconds. The average seizure duration is 72 seconds. Detailed description of this dataset is given in Table 4.2. The file format of the EEG time series in this dataset is. edf.

4.4.3 European Epileptic Dataset

There are 30 patients EEG recordings in the European Epilepsy-Database. The ages of the patients are between 13 and 67 years. In EEG data collection, the recordings are done with a 19-channel system based on the international 10–20 system channel configuration with referential montage. There are 276 seizures identified in the total 4604 hours of EEG recordings in the dataset. A summary of this dataset is provided in Table 4.3. The EEG time series are saved in .edf file format.

Table 4.3 Description of European Epileptic dataset

Patient no.	Gender	Age of patients in years	No. of recorded seizures
1	Male	36	11
2	Female	46	8
3	Male	41	8
4	Female	67	5
5	Female	52	8
6	Male	65	8
7	Male	36	5
8	Male	26	22
9	Male	47	6
10	Male	44	11
11	Male	48	14
12	Male	28	9
13	Male	46	8
14	Female	62	6
15	Female	41	5
16	Female	15	6
17	Female	17	9
18	Male	47	7
19	Male	32	22
20	Male	47	7
21	Female	31	8
22	Male	38	7
23	Male	50	9
24	Female	54	10
25	Male	42	8
26	Male	13	9
27	Male	58	9
28	Female	35	9
29	Male	50	10
30	Female	16	12
Total seizures			276

4.5 DATASET AVAILABILITY

To download the epilepsy datasets, please visit the following websites:

1. University of Bonn dataset (http://epileptologie-bonn.de/)
2. CHB-MIT dataset (https://www.physionet.org/pn6/chbmit/)
3. European Epilepsy dataset (http://epilepsy-database.eu/)

ACKNOWLEDGMENTS

The authors acknowledge the sources of public EEG epilepsy databases including CHB-MIT, University of Bonn, and University of Freiberg. The authors also thank the researchers involved in the studying of epileptic seizures in the Centre for Intelligent Signal and Imaging Research (CISIR).

REFERENCES

1. Bromfield E, Cavazos J, Sirven J. *An Introduction to Epilepsy [Internet]*. West Hartford: *American Epilepsy Society*; 2006.
2. Ben-Menachem E. Vagus-nerve stimulation for the treatment of epilepsy. *Lancet Neurol.* 2002;1(8):477–482.
3. Schachter SC, Saper CB. Vagus nerve stimulation. *Epilepsia.* 1998;39(7):677–686.
4. http://www.prophecypodcast.com/journal/2012/10/5/grand-mal-seizure.html.
5. Päivinen N, Lammi S, Pitkänen A, Nissinen J, Penttonen M, Grönfors T. Epileptic seizure detection: a nonlinear viewpoint. *Comput Methods Programs Biomed.* 2005;79(2):151–159.
6. Yuan Q, Zhou W, Liu Y, Wang J. Epileptic seizure detection with linear and nonlinear features. *Epilepsy Behav.* 2012;24(4):415–421.
7. Lee S-H, Lim JS, Kim J-K, Yang J, Lee Y. Classification of normal and epileptic seizure EEG signals using wavelet transform, phase-space reconstruction, and Euclidean distance. *Comput Methods Programs Biomed.* 2014;116(1):10–25.
8. Senhadji L, Wendling F. Epileptic transient detection: wavelets and time-frequency approaches. *Neurophysiol Clin Neurophysiol.* 2002;32(3):175–192.
9. Gotman J. Automatic seizure detection: improvements and evaluation. *Electroencephalogr Clin Neurophysiol.* 1990;76(4):317–324.
10. Adeli H, Zhou Z, Dadmehr N. Analysis of EEG records in an epileptic patient using wavelet transform. *J Neurosci Methods.* 2003;123(1):69–87.
11. Adeli H, Hung S-L. *Machine Learning: Neural Networks, Genetic Algorithms, and Fuzzy Systems*. New York: John Wiley & Sons, Inc; 1994.
12. Subasi A, Erçelebi E. Classification of EEG signals using neural network and logistic regression. *Comput Methods Programs Biomed.* 2005;78(2):87–99.
13. Subasi A. Automatic detection of epileptic seizure using dynamic fuzzy neural networks. *Expert Syst Appl.* 2006;31(2):320–328.
14. Guo L, Rivero D, Dorado J, Munteanu CR, Pazos A. Automatic feature extraction using genetic programming: an application to epileptic EEG classification. *Expert Syst Appl.* 2011;38(8):10425–10436.
15. Kumar Y, Dewal M, Anand R. Epileptic seizure detection using DWT based fuzzy approximate entropy and support vector machine. *Neurocomputing.* 2014;133: 271–279.
16. Tzallas AT, Tsipouras MG, Fotiadis DI. Epileptic seizure detection in EEGs using time–frequency analysis. *Inf Technol Biomed IEEE Trans.* 2009;13(5):703–710.
17. Das AB, Bhuiyan MIH, Alam SS. Classification of EEG signals using normal inverse Gaussian parameters in the dual-tree complex wavelet transform domain for seizure detection. *SIViP.* 2016;10(2):259–266.
18. Hosseini SA, Akbarzadeh-T M-R, Naghibi-Sistani M-B. Methodology for epilepsy and epileptic seizure recognition using chaos analysis of brain signals. *Intell Technol Techniques Pervas Comput.* 2013:20.
19. Hosseini SA, Akbarzadeh-T M, Naghibi-Sistani MB. Qualitative and quantitative evaluation of EEG signals in epileptic seizure recognition. *Int J Intell Syst Appl.* 2013;5(6):41.

20. Chen G. Automatic EEG seizure detection using dual-tree complex wavelet-Fourier features. *Expert Syst Appl*. 2014;41(5):2391–2394.

21. Xie S, Krishnan S. Wavelet-based sparse functional linear model with applications to EEGs seizure detection and epilepsy diagnosis. *Med Biol Eng Comput*. 2013;51(1–2):49–60.

22. Acharya UR, Sree SV, Ang PCA, Yanti R, Suri JS. Application of non-linear and wavelet based features for the automated identification of epileptic EEG signals. *Int J Neural Syst*. 2012;22(02).

23. Wang D, Miao D, Xie C. Best basis-based wavelet packet entropy feature extraction and hierarchical EEG classification for epileptic detection. *Expert Syst Appl*. 2011;38(11):14314–14320.

24. Upadhyay R, Jharia S, Padhy PK, Kankar PK. Application of wavelet fractal features for the automated detection of epileptic seizure using electroencephalogram signals. *Int J Biomed Eng Technol*. 2015;19(4):355–372.

25. Kumar A, Kolekar MH. Machine learning approach for epileptic seizure detection using wavelet analysis of EEG signals. *Paper presented at: Medical Imaging, m-Health and Emerging Communication Systems (MedCom), International Conference on*; 2014.

26. Kulasuriya K, Perera M. Forecasting epileptic seizures using EEG signals, wavelet transform and artificial neural networks. *Paper presented at: IT in Medicine and Education (ITME), International Symposium on*; 2011.

27. Bateman D. The future of neurology services in the UK. *Pract Neurol*. 2011;11(3):134–135.

28. Amin HU, Malik AS, Kamel N, Hussain M. A novel approach based on data redundancy for feature extraction of EEG signals. *Brain Topogr*. 2016;29(2):207–217.

29. Amin HU, Malik AS, Ahmad RF, et al. Feature extraction and classification for EEG signals using wavelet transform and machine learning techniques. *Australas Phys Eng Sci Med*. 2015;38(1):139–149.

30. Liu A, Hahn J, Heldt G, Coen R. Detection of neonatal seizures through computerized EEG analysis. *Electroencephalogr Clin Neurophysiol*. 1992;82(1):30–37.

31. Gotman J, Flanagan D, Rosenblatt B, Bye A, Mizrahi E. Evaluation of an automatic seizure detection method for the newborn EEG. *Electroencephalogr Clin Neurophysiol*. 1997;103(3):363–369.

32. Hassanpour H, Mesbah M, Boashash B. Time-frequency feature extraction of newborn EEG seizure using SVD-based techniques. *EURASIP J Appl Signal Process*. 2004:2544–2554. 2004.

33. Wilson SB, Scheuer ML, Emerson RG, Gabor AJ. Seizure detection: evaluation of the Reveal algorithm. *Clin Neurophysiol*. 2004;115(10):2280–2291.

34. Greene BR, Boylan GB, Reilly RB, de Chazal P, Connolly S. Combination of EEG and ECG for improved automatic neonatal seizure detection. *Clin Neurophysiol*. 2007;118(6):1348–1359.

35. Andrzejak RG, Lehnertz K, Mormann F, Rieke C, David P, Elger CE. Indications of nonlinear deterministic and finite-dimensional structures in time series of brain electrical activity: dependence on recording region and brain state. *Phys Rev E*. 2001;64(6):061907.

36. Goldberger AL, Amaral LAN, Glass L, et al. PhysioBank, PhysioToolkit, and PhysioNet: components of a new research resource for complex physiologic signals. *Circulation*. 2000;101(23):e215–e220.

37. Nasehi S, Pourghassem H. Epileptic seizure onset detection algorithm using dynamic cascade feed-forward neural networks. *Paper presented at: Intelligent Computation and Bio-Medical Instrumentation (ICBMI), International Conference on*; 2011.

CHAPTER 5

Alcohol Addiction

Contents

5.1 INTRODUCTION

According to the World Health Organization (WHO),[1] alcohol misuse is common among primary care patients, and results in considerable suffering, mortality, and economic costs (World Health Organization, 2011). Alcohol use is categorized as unsafe drinking if alcohol consumption exceeds 48 g per day or 144 g per week (Parsons and Nixon[2]). Drinking severity can be classified into heavy drinking, alcohol abuse (AA), and alcohol dependence (AD). Both AA and AD are described distinctly, according to the *Diagnostic and Statistical Manual of Mental Disorders IV* (DSM-IV),[3] as a severe form of alcohol drinking that causes distress or harm to drinker. As defined in the DSM-IV, AA is indicated as the recurring use of alcohol despite its negative consequences such as social, interpersonal, and legal problems. AD or alcoholism is the most severe form of alcohol use and is characterized by an increased tolerance and physical dependence on alcohol. People with AA and AD are referred to as alcohol abusers and alcoholics, respectively. In this study, the two DSM-IV disorders, AA and AD, will be referred to as alcohol use disorder (AUD).

Designing EEG Experiments for Studying the Brain.
DOI: http://dx.doi.org/10.1016/B978-0-12-811140-6.00005-9
© 2017 Elsevier Inc.
All rights reserved.

Screening and assessment of alcohol-related problems are mainly based on self-reports. For screening purposes, it has been concluded that only using self-reports is insufficient and there is a need to incorporate additional methods. In addition, accuracy of self-reporting has been questioned, especially for heavy drinkers, and people tended to underreport alcohol consumption quantity. Electroencephalography (EEG) is a brain imaging technique that can directly capture brain electrical voltage potentials over the scalp.[4] The variations in the brain electrical potentials reflecting the changes inside the brain neuronal networks occur due to any stimulation. The EEG can be analyzed using computational techniques to extract useful information for assessment of changes in neuronal networks.[4,5] It is reported that EEG has the potential to discriminate between alcoholics and control subjects.[6] Therefore, in this chapter we focus on the use of EEG to discriminate among AA, AD, and normal controls.

5.2 IMPORTANCE OF STUDYING DRUG ADDICTION

The treatment of alcohol abusers requires medical professionals to determine the existence of addiction by using addiction assessment techniques.[7] The assessment techniques answer questions such as whether an addiction exists, what is the extent of the addiction, and whether cooccurring conditions (mental disorders) exist. Once such information about a patient is clear, then the medical professionals try to take the best approach toward treating an individual's addiction issue. Initially, in the addiction assessment, the medical professionals involved the family members of the patient to seek drug and alcohol treatment. The addiction assessment enables medical professionals to understand the patient's situation and determine the most appropriate level of care and treatment.

In the addiction assessment process, many trained professionals are involved such as medical doctors, nurses, psychologists, therapists, and psychiatrists. The involvement of multiple professionals helps to ensure that the patient receives the most appropriate treatment. The assessment process is simple and straightforward. The clinicians use a standard screening tool (a questionnaire), which the patient needs to fill out by providing information regarding current alcohol use, health history, previous treatment history, symptoms, behavior, and the worst effects of the addiction on his/her life. The clinicians may ask for a face-to-face interview to understand the situation more clearly, while all the provided information is strictly confidential and used only for treatment purposes. There are standard screening questionnaire tools available such as the Alcohol Use Disorders

Identification Test (AUDIT), National Institute on Drug Use Screening Tool (NIDA), and CAGE questionnaire.[8–10] The CAGE contains four questions: (1) Have you ever felt you should *CUT* down on your drinking?; (2) Have others *ANNOYED* you by criticizing your drinking?; (3) Have you ever felt *GUILTY* about your drinking?; and (4) Have you ever felt the need to drink at *EYE* opening (in the morning)? The score of CAGE is between 0 and 1. Thus, two "yes" responses in the above questions will indicate the presence of addiction.[11] The AUDIT was developed for screening of alcohol abusers by the WHO in 1982. The AUDIT is a standard questionnaire that includes questions about the quantity and frequency of the alcohol use, dependence symptoms, and alcohol-related problems. It identifies patients who have problems with alcohol and who are dependent or not dependent.[12]

EEG- and event-related potential (ERP)-based screening tools are reported in literature. The EEG low-voltage alpha was associated with alcohol use disorders. It was observed that alcoholics were more likely to show low-voltage alpha than nonalcoholics.[13] Further, another study has shown that EEG can detect among alcohol patients to determine whether they relapsed or abstained from alcohol within 3 months after treatment.[13] The results suggested that the neural activity of those patients who relapsed was more desynchronized over the frontal regions, indicating functional disturbance in the prefrontal cortex. In addition, a 2016 study reported significant differences among alcohol abusers, alcoholics, and control subjects using EEG features with machine-learning techniques.[14] These studies indicated that the EEG technique has the potential to be used as a screening tool for the assessment of alcohol-addicted patients. The EEG enables the assessors to understand the neuronal behaviors of the patients and seek the most appropriate treatment.

5.3 PROBLEM FORMULATION

The problem here is the reliance of traditional screening methods using self-reports based on the honesty of patients. Alcoholic screening needs to be measured by another more reliable source to increase screening accuracy and verify the results of the self-report. Hence, this problem can be addressed by the research question: What is the quantitative difference in EEG signals between AUD patients and healthy people?

For this problem, it is hypothesized that AUD alters the function of the human brain and leads to the differences between problematic alcohol users and healthy people. The differences are more significant in alcohol-dependent patients than in alcohol abusers.

5.4 RESEARCH DESIGN

Participants who meet the DSM-IV criteria were enrolled for the experiments.[3] Participants were randomized and assigned into two separate groups (same sample size) with different drinking status:

- Control group (group of participants without the disease or just minor disease): participants who are evaluated as healthy normal people
- Case group (group of participants with the disease of interest): participants who are evaluated as AUD

The case group is then further assigned into two separate groups:

- Case 1: participants who are evaluated as alcohol abuse (AA)
- Case 2: participants who are evaluated as alcohol dependence (AD)

Based on the recruitment requirements previously mentioned, the experiment is defined as a case-control study with random samples. There are in total three independent samples and it is required to test the hypothesis based on the significant different power of each pair of two groups (control vs case 1 vs case 2) so the independent two samples' t-test is used for each pair of comparisons.

5.4.1 Hypothesis

Null hypothesis: the EEG spectral power is not different among groups (statistical null). *Biological aspect* means that chronic and heavy drinking does not have any effect on the brain activities (biological null).

Alternative hypothesis: the EEG spectral power is significantly different among groups (control, case 1, and case 2) and more significant between case 2 and control than between case 1 and control. This phenomenon indicates the alteration in the brain activities in AUD with more severity in alcoholics.

5.4.2 Sample Size Computation

Based on the hypothesis, EEG spectral power (absolute power or relative power) is selected as the test variable for sample size calculation; see Table 5.1. Because it is the measurement variable, the test is calculated and compared based on the mean value.

The convention in most biological research is to use a significance level $\alpha = 0.05$ ($Z_{\alpha/2} = 1.96$) and the power value $\beta = 80\%$ ($Z_{\beta} = 0.84$). This means that

- If the significant difference in mean power between two groups is larger than 5%, the null hypothesis can be rejected, or type I error.

Table 5.1 Sample size calculation

Reference	Notes	Alcoholics (n_1)	Controls (n_2)	Mean difference $(\mu_1 - \mu_2)$	Standard deviation (SD)	Effect size (ES)	Sample size (n)
Ehlers and Phillips[8]	Alpha power in P3	61	176	14.9	4.41	3.39	2
	Alpha power in P4	61	176	18.3	5.33	3.45	2

- If the significant difference in mean power between two groups is smaller than 20%, the null hypothesis can be considered again.

There is no more information for estimating so these values are chosen for the significant test.

Because two independent samples are compared with respect to continuous outcome and difference in mean variable, the sample size per group can be estimated by[15]:

$$n = \left[\frac{r+1}{r}\right]\left(\frac{Z_\beta + Z_{\alpha/2}}{\text{ES}}\right)^2$$

where r: ratio of controls to cases; $Z_{\alpha/2}$: represents the desired level of significant level; Z_β: represents the desired power; ES: effect size.

The effect size can be computed for groups with different sample size by adjusting the calculation of the pooled standard deviation with weights for the sample sizes. This adjustment is overall identical with d_{Cohen} or g_{Hedges} with a correction of a positive bias in the standard deviation.

$$\text{ES} = \frac{\mu_1 - \mu_2}{\text{SD}}$$

$$\text{SD} = \sqrt{\frac{(n_1 - 1)s_1^2 + (n_2 - 1)s_2^2}{n_1 + n_2 - 2}}$$

where μ_1, μ_2: mean values of case group and control group; n_1, n_2: sample size of case group and control group; s_1, s_2: standard deviation of case group and control group.

The authors found a previous study by Ehlers and Phillips[16] who investigated the association between alcohol dependence and EEG parameters. The mean and standard deviation of EEG alpha frequency at parietal sites P3 and P4 from the previous were used for sample size calculation. The calculated sample size is too small, i.e., sample size is 2 for one group or 6 for the total (3 groups). The reason is that there are huge differences between the mean of control and alcohol users of EEG alpha activity at parietal sites. Since the number 2 is quite small and the results of three groups with such a small number of participants may not be suitable for statistical test to compare results, the investigator recruited more participants in the study to be able to statistically verify the experimental results. Hence, 15 participants were recruited in the control group, as well as 18 alcoholic participants and 12 alcohol abusers.

5.4.3 Subjects Details

Data acquisition was performed at University Malaya Medical Center (UMMC) and Clinic Bingkor in Kota Kinabalu, Sabah, Malaysia from the following:

- 12 alcohol abusers (mean age 56.70 ± 15.33 years)
- 18 alcoholics (mean age 46.80 ± 9.29 years)
- 15 controls (mean age 42.67 ± 15.90 years)

The participants belonged to different ethnicities including Kadazan Dusun (Sabah, Malaysia), Indian (Malaysia), and Burmese.

The Alcohol Use Disorders Identification Test (AUDIT)[17] (see Appendix 5A) was performed by doctors and physicians at the University Malaya Centre of Addiction Sciences (UMCAS) to evaluate the drinking status of participants. According to their alcohol consumption, the participants were divided into two groups. They were grouped into controls if their alcohol consumption score (first three questions of AUDIT) was less than 4 and total AUDIT score was less than 8.[18] Otherwise, participants were grouped into AUDs if they had a total AUDIT score greater than 7. In addition, selection and diagnosis for alcoholics employed Mini International Neuropsychiatric Interview—MINI[19] (Appendix 5B) and Alcohol Withdrawal Assessment Scoring Guidelines—CIWA-Ar[20] (Appendix 5C). The selected participants were briefly introduced to the experiment design and were required to sign a consent form (Appendix 2C) before performing the EEG recording.

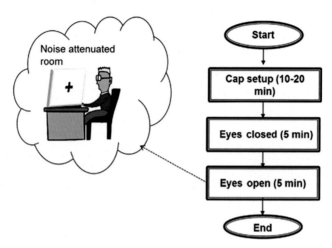

Figure 5.1 Experiment design.

5.5 EXPERIMENT PROCEDURE

The experiment design was approved by the local ethics committee at the University Malaya Medical Centre (UMMC). The experiment was designed as a single factorial study where the only interested factor manipulates AUD severity (healthy vs AUD) with two levels of physiological states, i.e., eyes closed (EC) and eyes open (EO), as depicted in Fig. 5.1.

Recording during each physiological condition lasted for 5 minutes, and was carried out in separate sessions with a 1-minute intersession break. The recordings were conducted in the morning in a sound-attenuated room to avoid interference with meal times and any other major disturbances. The process was divided into three steps:

- Step 1 was setting up the experiment using a 19-channel wearable cap. Proper caps were selected to fit participants' head size to ensure data quality. This process took about 10– 15 minutes.
- Step 2 was the eyes-closed (EC) session: patients were required to sit comfortably on a chair with eyes closed, awake, and with minimized movements.
- Step 3 was the eyes-open (EO) session: participants were required to concentrate on a black fixation point ("+") on a white computer screen in front of them with minimum of eyes movements or blinking.

For every EEG recording, participants had 1-minute break between each session and 1 extra minute at the beginning of the recording sessions to avoid unstable state.

5.6 SOFTWARE/HARDWARE DETAILS

Hardware details: Discovery 24E EEG and Enobio.

- Discovery system has 24 channels including 19 channels for data collection (FP1, FP2, F7, F3, Fz, F4, F8, T3, C3, Cz, C4, T4, T5, P3, Pz, P4, T6, O1, and O2), 1 channel for ground, 2 channels for reference, and 2 others for event timing. The electrode positions of the system were defined according to the international 10–20 system with amplitude unit in microvolts. Earlobe reference electrodes were used for all recordings. The ground electrode was placed above the nasion about 1/10 the distance from nasion to inion. Electrode impedance was maintained below $10\,\mathrm{k\Omega}$ by adding electrogel into electrodes using a syringe. DC amplifier and BrainMaster Discovery software were used for EEG recording.

- The second system, Enobio, is a wireless system with 19 data channels as found in the Discovery 24E EEG with one external input channel and two electrodes for mastoid references. Enobio system uses nanovolts as amplitude unit. Therefore, the recorded data had to be rescaled before further analysis.

In the BrainMaster system, the data were recorded with sampling rate of 512 samples per second and then filtered and reconstructed at 256 samples per second. EEG signals were filtered by the amplifier with bandwidth about 0.1–100 Hz. The data were then transferred to PC through an optically and magnetically isolated USB cable. For the Enobio system, the signals were transmitted through Bluetooth protocol at sampling rate of 500 samples per second. EEG signals of both systems were saved in .edf format.

To make the data compatible between the two EEG systems, data recorded from Enobio were first converted to microvolt unit by multiplying by 1000. Nineteen channels from both systems were rearranged in the same order and used for further processing. All signals were resampled to 256 samples per second and rereferenced using common average reference (CAR).[21]

$$V_i^{\mathrm{CAR}} = V_i^{\mathrm{ER}} - \frac{1}{n}\sum_{j=1}^{n} V_j^{\mathrm{ER}}$$

where V_i^{ER} was the potential between the ith electrode and the reference and n was the number of electrodes in the montage (i.e., 19 in this study). Selecting CAR as reference also helped to maximize the signal-to-noise ratio. CAR was also easy to implement and was considered to be superior to the ear reference method.[21]

Artifacts due to eye movements, blinks, or muscle activity and drowsiness were semiautomatically detected using NeuroGuide software. This included a selection of 60 seconds of artifact-free epochs from the raw data. In the software, the selected EEG segments were also estimated for reliability using the split-half reliability score (SHR score). SHR is the ratio of variance between the odd and even time points of the time series from the selected EEG. The selection was performed with SHR score > 0.90. Artifact-free EEG data was then applied to custom MATLAB scripts for further analysis.

5.7 DATA DESCRIPTION

This section provides description of the physiological data and subjective data collected during the experimentation.

5.7.1 Experiment Data Accompanying This Chapter

EEG and ECG raw data for one subject are provided with this book. The details of these files are provided in Table 5.2. To access these EEG files, please go to the directory BookData\Chap05\EEG in the data files accompanying this book. For the complete dataset of 40 subjects, please contact the authors at brainexpbook@gmail.com.

5.8 RELEVANT PAPERS

This section provides a list of some of the papers that have utilized the data acquired from the experiment described in this chapter. The

Table 5.2 EEG data description

S. No.	EEG condition	Description
1	Eyes closed	Five minutes EEG recording during resting state eyes-closed condition.
2	Eyes open	Five minutes EEG recording during resting state eyes-open condition.

following journal paper should be cited when using the experiment design or the data provided with this chapter.

- Mumtaz W, Vuong PL, Xia L, Malik AS, Rashid RBA. Automatic diagnosis of alcohol use disorder using EEG features. *Knowledge-Based Syst*; 2016. doi:10.1016/j.knosys.2016.04.026.

ACKNOWLEDGMENTS

This chapter provides the details of the experiment design available in the paper mentioned in Section 5.8 and in the MS thesis of Pham Voung, which is available at Universiti Teknologi PETRONAS.

REFERENCES

1. WHO. <http://www.who.int/substance_abuse/publications/global_alcohol_report/en/>. Accessed October 30, 2014.
2. Parsons OA, Nixon SJ. Cognitive functioning in sober social drinkers: a review of the research since 1986. *J Stud Alcohol*. 1998;59(2):180–190.
3. Spitzer RL, Gibbon ME, Skodol AE, Williams JB, First MB. *DSM-IV casebook: a learning companion to the diagnostic and statistical manual of mental disorders*. 4th ed. Arlington, VA: American Psychiatric Association; 1994.
4. Amin HU, Malik AS, Ahmad RF, et al. Feature extraction and classification for EEG signals using wavelet transform and machine learning techniques. *Australas Phys Eng Sci Med*. 2015;38(1):139–149.
5. Amin HU, Malik AS, Kamel N, Hussain M. A novel approach based on data redundancy for feature extraction of EEG signals. *Brain Topogr*. 2016;29(2):207–217.
6. Acharya UR, Sree SV, Chattopadhyay S, Suri JS. Automated diagnosis of normal and alcoholic EEG signals. *Int J Neural Syst*. 2012;22(03):1250011.
7. Samet S, Waxman R, Hatzenbuehler M, Hasin DS. Assessing addiction: concepts and instruments. *Addict Sci Clin Pract*. 2007;4(1):19–31.
8. Bohn MJ, Babor TF, Kranzler HR. The Alcohol Use Disorders Identification Test (AUDIT): validation of a screening instrument for use in medical settings. *J Stud Alcohol*. 1995;56(4):423–432.
9. Bergman H, Källmén H. Alcohol use among Swedes and a psychometric evaluation of the alcohol use disorders identification test. *Alcohol Alcohol*. 2002;37(3):245–251.
10. Bradley KA, Bush KR, Epler AJ, et al. Two brief alcohol-screening tests from the Alcohol Use Disorders Identification Test (AUDIT): validation in a female Veterans Affairs patient population. *Arch Intern Med*. 2003;163(7):821–829.
11. NIAAA. Alcohol Alert. 2005; <http://pubs.niaaa.nih.gov/publications/aa65/AA65.htm>. Accessed September 31, 2016.
12. Higgins-Biddle JC, Babor TF, WHO. Brief intervention for hazardous and harmful drinking: a manual for use in primary care; 2001.
13. Winterer G, Klöppel B, Heinz A, et al. Quantitative EEG (QEEG) predicts relapse in patients with chronic alcoholism and points to a frontally pronounced cerebral disturbance. *Psychiatry Res*. 1998;78(1–2):101–113.
14. Mumtaz W, Vuong PL, Xia L, Malik AS, Rashid RBA. Automatic diagnosis of alcohol use disorder using EEG features. *Knowledge-Based Syst*. 2016;105:48–59.

15. Sathian B, Sreedharan J, Baboo SN, Sharan K, Abhilash E, Rajesh E. Relevance of sample size determination in medical research. *Nepal J Epidemiol.* 2010;1(1):4–10.
16. Ehlers CL, Phillips E. Association of EEG alpha variants and alpha power with alcohol dependence in Mexican American young adults. *Alcohol.* 2007;41(1):13–20.
17. Reinert DF, Allen JP. The alcohol use disorders identification test: an update of research findings. *Alcohol Clin Exp Res.* 2007;31(2):185–199.
18. Bush K, Kivlahan DR, McDonell MB, Fihn SD, Bradley KA. The AUDIT alcohol consumption questions (AUDIT-C): an effective brief screening test for problem drinking. *Arch Intern Med.* 1998;158(16):1789–1795.
19. Amorim P. Mini International Neuropsychiatric Interview (MINI): validação de entrevista breve para diagnóstico de transtornos mentais. *Rev Bras Psiquiatr.* 2000;22(3):106–115.
20. Sullivan JT, Sykora K, Schneiderman J, Naranjo CA, Sellers EM. Assessment of alcohol withdrawal: the revised clinical institute withdrawal assessment for alcohol scale (CIWA-Ar). *Br J Addict.* 1989;84(11):1353–1357.
21. McFarland DJ, McCane LM, David SV, Wolpaw JR. Spatial filter selection for EEG-based communication. *Electroencephalogr Clin Neurophysiol.* 1997;103(3):386–394.

CHAPTER 6

Passive Polarized and Active Shutter 3D TVs

Contents

6.1 INTRODUCTION

Three-dimensional (3D) technology is now popular in the entertainment industry, especially in the production of movies, 3D video games, and 3D-based television broadcasting. This phenomenal progress started growing rapidly after the successful launch of the 3D movie *Avatar* in 2009 by James Cameron. *Avatar* created a wide awareness in public about watching 3D movies and dramatically increased 3D-based film production. In 2015, *Jurassic World* earned $205 million in 3D theaters outside the United States, reflecting the popularity of 3D movies worldwide. As of 2016, an increasing number of newly released movies have a 3D version, which reflects public acceptance of 3D technology. Filmmakers and cinemas are

Designing EEG Experiments for Studying the Brain.
DOI: http://dx.doi.org/10.1016/B978-0-12-811140-6.00006-0

© 2017 Elsevier Inc.
All rights reserved.

continuing their investments in 3D movies to attract more viewers and earn more revenue.

Despite the fact that 3D technology is rapidly growing, there are concerns about the side effects of 3D contents on viewers' visual and cognitive systems.[1] Viewers reported that they experienced discomfort when watching 3D movies in the cinema.[2] The most common types of discomfort include dizziness, headaches, nausea, and visual strain.[3] In addition to that, there had been cases where some of the viewers claimed that they could not fully enjoy the 3D movies due to the fact that while watching 3D movie, the feeling of 3D depth perception was not continuous, i.e., the viewers can see in 3D for a moment followed by a feeling of seeing in 2D and then again in 3D, etc.

Previously, most research had studied the effects of 3D viewing from the ergonomic perspective, mainly assessed based on the psychological effects that can be experienced as symptoms of gastrointestinal distress (i.e., stomach ache), disorientation (i.e., postural instability), or visual symptoms of eyestrain or eye fatigue.[4] Initially, the evaluation of the effects was conducted based on participative measures such as questionnaires, interviews, and user feedback ratings based on the quality of the perceived 3D stimuli.[5-8] Few studies have employed quantitative methods to measure visual and mental fatigue.[9-12] It is reported that some symptoms of viewers' discomfort have been linked with the characteristics of visual scene stimuli and are due to accommodative and vergence stress.[7,13]

In addition to that, the type of 3D display technologies used for watching 3D stereoscopic content may cause visual fatigue.[14] For instance, the liquid crystal shutter glasses used in 3D active shutter systems may induce the sensation of flickering (liquid crystal shutters), while the color filter glasses technology may cause binocular rivalry (color filter glasses). Other 3D technologies like head-mounted displays (HMDs) may cause eyestrain because of optical misalignments and display features.[15,16]

However, the impression of watching 3D content depends on the quality of 3D display screens and the underlying 3D technology used by the manufacturers. In other words, the level of comfort during 3D presentation for the viewers directly depends on the quality of 3D display technologies. Thus, 3D display devices should provide high-quality 3D depth perception to the viewers without any viewing complaints.

In general, a 3D display would provide additional information of sense of depth to the viewers as compared to traditional 2D display devices; it is likely that the former is closer to human binocular vision. Ideally, viewers should feel high satisfaction in 3D mode as compared to 2D mode rather than reporting viewing complaints. This gives rise to the question: What is the main cause of viewers' dissatisfaction in watching 3D content? Therefore, the aim of this study was to study the effects of two common consumer 3DTV technologies on viewers' visual discomfort, and/or any other complaints such as visual fatigue, cognitive load, and aftereffects on vision, using physiological signals.

6.2 IMPORTANCE OF STUDYING 3D DISPLAY TECHNOLOGIES

Stereoscopic 3D technology is rapidly growing and has become famous not only in the entertainment market, but has also been adopted in the home in the form of 3D HDTVs, 3D cameras, 3D game players, 3D projectors, and 3D PCs. There are many different potential applications of 3D technology, such as real-time 3D simulation (used for education, training, experimentation, and human behaviors), virtual reality, architecture, 3D marketing, 3D video, and serious games. 3D technology may expand into a wider range of electronics in the future, to provide 3D webcams, photo frames, portable Blu-ray players, and much more for 3D TV channels.

In the market, two widely accepted and well-known 3D display technologies are available for home users, i.e., 3D passive polarized and 3D active shuttered technologies. Regardless of the fact that 3D display technology has made entertainment more interesting, especially watching action movies or playing video games, there has been concern from the end users about the expected side effects of 3D viewing. The reason is that 3D technology takes advantage of human binocular vision and creates 3D depth illusion and viewers feel the contents differently. Thus, researchers collected the feedback of the viewers and reported their complaints.[17,18] The most commonly reported complaints are 3D cross talk,[19] comfort/discomfort,[20,21] cognitive and visual fatigues,[14,22] motion sickness,[23] aftereffects,[3] and 3D effects on vision.[24]

Thus, the comparison of these two technologies is of wide interest to end users, i.e., which 3D type should be selected for home usage. The existing studies compared the two types using viewer feedback, having viewers fill out a questionnaire after being exposed to video content using these two 3D types. Thus, after reviewing the recent research studies, the following main points are extracted from their findings.[25–31]

- The quality of viewing of active shuttered 3D technology is better than passive polarized 3D technology, but viewers experience higher fidelity and brightness in active shuttered technology than in the passive polarized technology.

- The readability (e.g., reading small font) in the shuttered technology is superior to that of the polarized technology.
- Shuttered 3D provides more flickering than polarized 3D as reported by the participants. Hence, the flickering may induce more side effects for shuttered 3D such as eye fatigue, headache, and flash effect.

The viewers' feedback indirectly expresses their perception during watching the 3D content, either passive or active 3D. However, the subjective methods for quality assessment of 3D types could not explain the impact on the brain, i.e., the behavior of the actual neuronal mechanism that is involved in the processing of 3D visual information through the visual system, attentional and working memory resources, and the brain pathways. The study of the brain neuronal activities could explain the impact of watching the 3D content and the differences between the two 3D types.[26]

Although much research has been done on the ergonomic effects on exposure to stereoscopic display, understanding its impact on the human brain is somewhat incomplete. Early researchers have attempted to understand how the brain perceives depth perception in 3D especially with regards to our stereoscopic vision.[26] The vision research studies reported that there are specialized brain cells in the visual cortex that process the disparity-related information from the two images viewed by each eye in order to get depth information in the scene.[32–35] But the issue is that most research was limited to the visual cortex, while other connected regions of the brain that play a role in the handling of the 3D information are still not very clear.

Electroencephalography (EEG) is the most appropriate neuroimaging method to use for long duration while watching 3D videos or playing 3D games, as it is noninvasive and portable. Further, the time resolution of EEG is quite good, so the fast information processing of the brain that brings changes in the neuronal activity could be better understood. Hence, the motivation of the experiment described in this chapter is to compare the two 3D display types and explore the impact of viewing 3D on neuronal activity using EEG.

6.3 PROBLEM STATEMENT

Even though a considerable amount of research has been performed to investigate the ergonomic effects on the exposure to stereoscopic display, knowledge about its impact on human brain is relatively limited. Previous studies of the human brain explored the mechanism of depth perception and binocular vision ability, especially the visual system and disparity.[36–39] Furthermore, since much research focused on studying the human visual performance in the visual cortex, the roles played by other brain regions during stereoscopic vision are still poorly defined.

In addition to that, participative measures such as questionnaire and user feedback ratings have been widely employed to determine the level of visual discomfort in viewers. Nevertheless, a standard procedure, either a questionnaire or observation that is sensitive and robust in defining the level of visual discomfort of stereoscopic displays, has not yet been well recognized.[7] Besides that, the types of 3D stimuli used in some studies were designed to induce side effects (i.e., motion sickness, stress, etc.) or required the participants to be engaged in tasks such as playing 3D video games.

As the general aim is to assess the effects of 3D viewing, the type of 3D display plays an important role as the quality of experience depends on the performance of the display. In the past, the types of the 3D technology used in the studies were mainly commercial cinema 3D projectors and constructed 3D displays (in lab settings). While the former is not properly controlled (i.e., presence of noise, interaction between participants, etc.), the natural 3D viewing settings are compromised in the latter. As 3DTV display technology is relatively new, little work has been done in investigating the viewing effects due to the consumer grade 3DTV displays, hence knowledge about the effects of viewing based on these technologies is also limited. The following research questions were investigated in this experiment:

Q1: What are the physiological effects due to stereoscopic 3DTV (active shutter and passive polarized) viewing?

Q2: Which stereoscopic 3DTV viewing improves cognitive performances (i.e., enhanced working memory and attentional level) in viewers?

The first research question (Q1) is concerned with the physiological effects of visualizing videos via stereoscopic 3DTV, which are measured using the electrophysiological signals (EEG and ECG). EEG signals capture brain voltage potentials that can be analyzed using computational techniques to extract useful information for assessment of brain cognitive states.[40,41] ECG signals represent the dynamics of time interval between heartbeats.[42] ECG signals can be analyzed to determine the heart rate variability (HRV), which may reveal the changes in heartbeats due to suffering from visual or cognitive fatigues.

In the second question (Q2), the type of viewing technology that provides optimum visualization is determined based on the performance of working memory and visual attention, as well as HRV. The 3DTV provides more visual information along with depth perception and the fact that all sensory and cognitive information is processed in the brain; therefore, the changes in the brain activity could reflect the effects of viewing stereoscopic content.

6.4 SOFTWARE AND HARDWARE TOOLS

The list of equipment and software used in this experiment is described in Table 6.1.

Table 6.1 Description of hardware (equipment) and software

S. No.	Equipment	Description
01	Discovery 24E (hardware)	1. 1—Discovery 24E 2. 1—USB cable w/chokes (3 m) 3. 1—Two input channel cable★ 4. 1—BrainMaster carrying case ★for peripheral use only—Channel 23 and 24 (i.e., ECG, EMG)
02	Checktrode electrode tester	1—Checktrode electrode tester 2—9V battery supply
03	Gold disk electrodes (length: 1.2 m, female jack)	7 packs (5 electrodes/pack) = 35 electrodes

(*Continued*)

Table 6.1 Description of hardware (equipment) and software (Continued)

S. No.	Equipment	Description
04	Ear-clip electrode (gold disk, 1.2 m, female jack)	1 pair (1 black, 1 white) = 2 electrodes ★to be used with gold electrodes only
05	Electro caps (19—tin electrodes)	4 sizes: 1. 1—Small (50–54 cm) 2. 1—Medium/small (52–56 cm) 3. 1—Large/medium (56–60 cm) 4. 1—Large (58–62)
06	Ear-clip electrodes (tin disk, 1.2 m, female jack)	★to be used only with electro caps/electrodes of the same metal type (tin)
07	Ten20 conductive paste (for single electrodes)	1. 1—4oz 10/20 paste (3-pack) 2. 1—4oz 10/20 paste jar
08	NuPrep (skin prep gel)	1 box of 6-pack tubes

(Continued)

Table 6.1 Description of hardware (equipment) and software (Continued)

S. No.	Equipment	Description
09	Electro-Gel (for electro caps)	473 mL Electro-Gel
10	Disposable sponge disks	2 packs
11	Measuring tape	2 units
12	Marking pencil	1 unit
13	Syringe *for Electro-Gel	2 units
14	Toothbrush *for cleaning electrodes	1 unit
15	NeuroGuide (Applied Neuroscience Inc.)	Version 2.7.2.0
16	MATLAB (MathWorks Inc.)	Version 2012a
17	Discovery 24E (BrainMaster)	Version 3.0
18	Toshiba laptop	Intel Core i7-720QM processor (6M cache, 1.6 GHz) and 500 GB
19	Sony 40-inch 3DTV	Sony 3D active shutter glasses, refresh rate 240 Hz, LED display, 1080p resolution, HDMI and USB slots
20	LG 42-inch 3DTV	LG passive polarized 3D technology display

6.5 EXPERIMENTAL DESIGN AND PROTOCOL

This section describes the experiment design protocol of this study including participant information, inclusion and exclusion criteria, sample size computation, and stimuli design.

6.5.1 Target Population

In this study, students on the university campus were the target population. All the students on the university campus were the entire set of units for which the findings of the research had been generalized. Three levels of students were studying on the campus, i.e., foundation level, undergraduate level, and postgraduate level. Equal opportunity to become a participant was given to all students who met the inclusion criteria.

6.5.2 Inclusion Criteria

- Participant must be a student at Universiti Teknologi PETRONAS
- Participant age should be between 18 and 25 years of age
- Participant must be physically and mentally healthy

6.5.3 Exclusion Criteria

The exclusion criteria are the requirements used for exclusion of participants from this study. In this study, participants are excluded when fail to provide written consent (Appendix 2C).

6.5.4 Sample Size Computation

The sample size computation for this study was not predefined because it was a pilot study. Further research on this topic may be required to properly compute the sample size using the mean differences among the three groups in this study, which are reported in the published papers. Please see the published papers in Section 6.7 in this chapter.

6.5.5 Participant Recruitment

In this study, 40 volunteers were recruited who were healthy university students (30 males and 10 females) aged between 19 and 25 years old (21.55 ± 1.52). The participants had normal or corrected-to-normal vision and had no neurophysiological impairments. As part of the inclusion criteria for participant recruitment, all recruited participants reported that they had normal vision and no medical history existed, and all had past experience in 3D viewing. However, those who reported that they had experienced severe visual discomfort during 3D viewing in the past, such as motion sickness, headache, and nausea, were excluded from the study. The target population was the undergraduate and postgraduate students of Universiti Teknologi PETRONAS (UTP). All the participants were informed about the experimental procedures and they provided a written Participant Information and Consent Form (see Appendix 2C). The protocol of this study was approved by the UTP Ethics Coordination Committee.

Participants were randomly divided into two equal groups (either 3D Active First or 3D Passive First). All participants in this study had an experience in 3D viewing (i.e., had watched 3D movies or played 3D games in the past). The demographic data including age, gender, and handedness of both experimental groups is listed in Appendix 6A.

6.5.6 Stimuli

Participants were exposed to a series of short video clips for 20 minutes in all three experimental conditions, i.e., 2D mode, 3D active mode, and 3D passive mode. However, the auditory stimulus was also present during the experiment but was kept at a very minimum volume. The inclusion of minimal auditory information was necessary in order to replicate the cinematic experience (but in a controlled setting) and it was also to prevent the viewers from feeling bored and drowsy over time.

In this experiment, a set of short video clips was used as the stimuli. The video clips were produced by Sony ("Sony Blu-Ray 3D Experience 2010, volume 2"), which was commercially available and contained good quality 3D content. The video clips were selected from the recommended imaginary animated and natural movies. Although different video clips may result in different brain and heart responses, the content of the video clips was not the main concern, since the same video clips were employed for 2D, 3DA (3D active shutter glasses), and 3DP (3D passive polarized glasses) viewing. Hence, the corresponding responses in each viewing mode can be observed by computing the difference between viewing modes. The description of all the video clips is summarized in Table 6.2.

6.5.7 Experiment Design

In this research, two sets of experiments were conducted to study different complaints reported by viewers about 3D content, through consumer 3D technologies on brain oscillations and heart responses. The first experiment was to investigate the difference in viewers' responses when viewing the stimuli on the 2D and the 3D displays (i.e., 3D active and 3D passive). As for the second experiment, the differences in the viewers' responses between 3D active viewing and 3D passive viewing were observed.

The participants were randomly divided into two groups: 3D Active First and 3D Passive First. The flows of the experiment for both groups are illustrated in Fig. 6.1. The 3D Active First group watched the clips first in a 3D active mode, followed by 3D passive, while the 3D Passive First watched the clips in 3D passive first and then in 3D active mode. This division of participants into two groups avoided the content novelty and practice effect in the experiment, which may cause biased effects on the results.

6.5.8 Experiment Procedure

The recording of EEG and ECG data took place during the resting states (i.e., eyes closed and eyes open) and the visual stimulation sessions (i.e.,

Table 6.2 Description of video clips in order of presentation

S. No.	Title of clip	Time (min)	Details
1	*A Christmas Carol* (Disney, 2009)	4.25	In this clip, Scrooge met the Ghost of Christmas Past. They flew together and Scrooge was brought back to his own past as a child.
2	*The Nightmare Before Christmas* (Disney, 2011)	2.20	This clip shows Jack sharing his ideas about the Christmas celebration with the Halloween Town residents. In a church hall, the monsters and ghosts were singing.
3	*Alice in Wonderland* (Disney, 2010)	2.11	Alice ran away to catch a white rabbit and reached a place named Wonderland. There she found the Hatter; later, the Red Queen's soldier seized him. Alice planned to escape and struggled to release the Hatter, so she presented herself as a guest and went to the Red Queen's castle.
4	*Toy Story 3* (Disney Pixar, 2010)	3.11	This clip shows Andy when he was little playing with his toys (a flashback). All of his toys were mistakenly placed in the garbage when he went to college. All the toys escaped and left Andy's house and reached the Sunnyside nursery.
5	*G-Force* (Disney, 2009)	3.28	In this scene, a race between the G-Force team and the FBI agents is presented. It is presented that one of the FBI cars became stuck while the other crashed because of fireworks during the chase.
6	*3D Sony Aquarium* (Sony PLC, 2010)	4.13	This clips shows a scene of a school of swimming fish and a bear diving into the aquarium.

2D and 3D). The recording begins with the eyes-closed session. The participants were instructed to sit as relaxed as they could while they were awake. Then the participants were instructed to focus on a black fixation point displayed at the center of a white screen so that the gaze was fixed during eyes-open recording. The eyes-closed session was conducted only once, i.e., at the very beginning of the experiment, while the eyes-open sessions were done prior to each visual stimulation session.

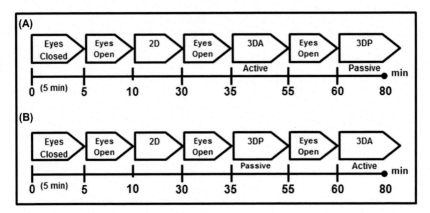

Figure 6.1 EEG recording flow diagram. (A) 3D active first group. (B) 3D passive first group.

As mentioned earlier, the visual stimulation session contained three conditions: 2D, 3DA, and 3DP. The stereoscopic 3D system requires viewing glasses, hence all participants wore a set of passive polarized glasses and active shutter glasses during 3DP and 3DA modes, respectively. However, no glasses were needed for the 2D viewing. The viewing glasses are only required during the 3D viewing modes, therefore the glasses were removed during the resting conditions and the breaks between sessions.

In addition, the participants were also instructed to minimize any physical movement as much as possible. After each recording session, they were given a 5–10 minute break, and no recording was involved during this period to allow them to rest; this also reduced the potential fatigue and drowsiness effect. However, during this time, they were asked to report their viewing experience by filling up the simulator sickness questionnaire (SSQ) (Appendix 5B). Prior to the viewing in other modes, the participants were required to perform the eyes-open test again to remove the transient effects that may be induced by the various video clips in the previous viewing sessions.

6.5.9 Self-Report Measures

In this experiment, the participants filled out the feedback form and thus subjective data was collected at the end of the experiment. The subjective data contained the user's 3D experience and responses against the standard SSQ and the feedback form. These questionnaires can be seen in Appendix 6B.

Table 6.3 SSQ Scores distribution

S. No.	Symptom	Nausea[a]	Oculomotor[b]	Disorientation[c]
1	General discomfort	1	1	0
2	Fatigue	0	1	0
3	Headache	0	1	0
4	Eyestrain	0	1	0
5	Difficulty focusing	0	1	1
6	Increased salivation	1	0	0
7	Sweating	1	0	0
8	Nausea	1	0	1
9	Difficulty concentrating	1	1	0
10	Fullness of head	0	0	1
11	Blurred vision	0	1	1
12	Dizziness with eyes open	0	0	1
13	Dizziness with eyes closed	0	0	1
14	Vertigo	0	0	1
15	Stomach awareness	1	0	0
16	Burping	1	0	0

Total SSQ score = $(A + B + C) \times 3.74$.
Scale multiplication factor:
[a]Nausea: $A = \text{score} \times 9.54$
[b]Oculomotor: $B = \text{score} \times 7.58$
[c]Disorientation: $C = \text{score} \times 13.92$

6.5.9.1 Simulator Sickness Questionnaire

The SSQ was filled out by all the participants regarding their experience during watching video clips in the three visual stimulation conditions. The SSQ standard was initially developed by Kennedy,[43] for the purpose of quantifying the symptoms experienced by viewers. The SSQ standard contained three main components: nausea, disorientation, and oculomotor problems. The general symptoms with their weightings are listed in Table 6.3 and an SSQ sample is provided in Appendix 6B.

The participants need to select one of four categories—None, Slight, Moderate, or Severe—and report the degree to which they experienced each of the symptoms. The quantity values for these scales are 0, 1, 2, and 3, respectively. The scale for each column was computed by multiplying the reported value of the symptom to the weight in each column and then summed down the column. The overall total SSQ score was determined by multiplying the sum of scores across the three columns with 3.74. The procedure for computing the column score is provided at the end of Table 6.3.

Table 6.4 EEG data description

S. No.	Directory name	EEG and ECG description
01	EC	This directory contains the baseline recording: 5 min for eyes–closed condition before watching any movie.
02	EO 2D	Baseline recording: 5 min for eyes–open condition before watching any movie.
03	2D	This directory contains EEG or ECG recording for 10 min during watching movie in 2D display mode. There were six clips presented to participants in 2D mode, hence the directory contains six files in .edf format.
04	EO 3DA	Baseline recording: 5 min for eyes–open condition after watching the movie in 2D display and before watching movie in 3D active display mode.
05	3DA	EEG or ECG recording for 10 min during watching movie in 3D active display mode. There were six clips presented to participants in 3DA mode, hence the directory contains six files in .edf format.
06	EO 3DP	Baseline recording: 5 min for eyes–open condition after watching the movie in 3D active display and before watching movie in 3D passive display mode.
07	3DP	EEG or ECG recording for 10 min during watching movie in 3D passive display mode. There were six clips presented to participants in 3DP mode, hence the directory contains six files in .edf format.

6.5.9.2 Subjective Data

The participants filled out a questionnaire about their self-preferences toward the available consumer 3D technologies (see Appendix 6B).

6.6 DATA DESCRIPTION

This section provides a description of the physiological data and subjective data collected during the experimentation.

6.6.1 Experiment Data Accompanying this Chapter

EEG and ECG raw data for one subject are provided with this book. The details of these files are provided in Table 6.4. To access these EEG or ECG

Table 6.5 SSQ and feedback questionnaire data

S. No.	File name	Description
01	ssq.xls	SSQ responses recorded after visualization of movie on 3D display modes (3D active and 3D passive).
02	fb.xls	At the end of the experiment, this feedback questionnaire was used to record the user self-preferences on 3D display technologies.

files, please go to the directory BookData\Chap06\EEG or BookData\Chap06\ECG in the data files accompanying this book. For the complete dataset of 40 subjects, please contact the authors at brainexpbook@gmail.com.

6.6.2 Questionnaire Data

The SSQ (SSQ questionnaire data) and user feedback on self-preference and feedback responses of one subject are provided in Table 6.5. To access these excel files, please go to the directory BookData\Chap06\Questionnaire Data.

6.7 RELEVANT PAPERS

This section provides a list of some of the papers that have utilized the data acquired from the experiment described in this chapter. The following papers should be cited when using the experiment design or the data provided with this chapter.

1. Malik AS, Khairuddin RNHR, Amin HU, Smith ML, Kamel N, Abdullah JM, Fawzy SM, Shim S. EEG based evaluation of stereoscopic 3D displays for viewer discomfort. *BioMed Eng OnLine*. 2015; 14:21.
2. Khairuddin HR, Malik AS, Mumtaz W, Kamel N, Xia L. Analysis of EEG signals regularity in adults during video game play in 2D and 3D. In: *Engineering in Medicine and Biology Society (EMBC), 2013 35th Annual International Conference of the IEEE*; 2013, pp. 2064–2067.

ACKNOWLEDGMENTS

This chapter provides the details of the experiment design available in the papers mentioned in Section 6.7 and in the MS thesis of Raja Nur Hamizah, which is available at Universiti Teknologi PETRONAS.

REFERENCES

1. Amin HU, Malik AS, Mumtaz W, Badruddin N, Kamel N. Evaluation of passive polarized stereoscopic 3D display for visual & mental fatigues. *Paper presented at: Engineering in Medicine and Biology Society (EMBC), 2015 37th Annual International Conference of the IEEE;* August 25–29, 2015.
2. Williams C. 3D films, TV and video games "cause nausea and headaches." *The Telegraph* 2011; <http://www.telegraph.co.uk/technology/8272497/3D-films-TV-and-video-games-cause-nausea-and-headaches.html>. Accessed November 2012.
3. Solimini AG. Are there side effects to watching 3D movies? A prospective crossover observational study on visually induced motion sickness. *PloS one.* 2013;8(2):e56160.
4. Skrandies W. Assessment of depth perception using psychophysical thresholds and stereoscopically evoked brain activity. *Doc Ophthalmol Adv Ophthalmol.* 2009;119(3):209–216.
5. Yano S, Ide S, Mitsuhashi T, Thwaites H. A study of visual fatigue and visual comfort for 3D HDTV/HDTV images. *Displays.* 2002;23:11.
6. Kooi FL, Toet A. Visual comfort of binocular and 3D displays. *Displays.* 2004;25:99–108.
7. Lambooij M, IJsselsteijn W. Visual discomfort and visual fatigue of stereoscopic displays: a review. *J Imaging Sci Technol.* 2009;53(3):1–14.
8. Pölönen M, Järvenpää T, Bilcu B. Stereoscopic 3D entertainment and its effect on viewing comfort: comparison of children and adults. *Appl Ergon.* 2013;44:151–160.
9. Y. Tran Wijesuryia N, Thuraisingham RA, Craig A, Nguyen HT. Increase in regularity and decrease in variability seen in EEG signals from alert to fatigue during a driving simulated task. *Paper presented at: 30th Annual International IEEE EMBS Conference;* August 20–24, 2008. Vancouver, British Columbia, Canada; 2008.
10. Li H-CO, Seo J, Kham K, Lee S. Measurement of 3D visual fatigue using event-related potential (ERP)—3D oddball paradigm. *3DTV Conference: The True Vision—Capture, Transmission and Display of 3D Video;* May 28–30, 2008. Istanbul, Turkey; 2008.
11. Muna S, Park M-C, Park S, Whang M. SSVEP and ERP measurement of cognitive fatigue caused by stereoscopic 3D. *Neurosci Lett.* 2012;525:89–94.
12. Amin HU, Malik AS, Badruddin N, Kamel N, Hussain M. Effects of stereoscopic 3D display technology on event-related potentials (ERPs). *Paper presented at: Neural Engineering (NER), 2015 7th International IEEE/EMBS Conference;* April 22–24, 2015.
13. Lambooij M, IJsselsteijn WA, Heynderickx I. Visual discomfort of 3D TV—assessment methods and modeling. *Displays.* 2011;32:209–218.
14. Ukai K, Howarth PA. Visual fatigue caused by viewing stereoscopic motion images: background, theories, and observations. *Displays.* 2008;29(2):106–116.
15. Kuze J, Ukai K. Subjective evaluation of visual fatigue caused by motion images. *Displays.* 2008;29(2):159–166.
16. Pölönen M, Salmimaa M, Takatalo J, Häkkinen J. Subjective experiences of watching stereoscopic Avatar and U2 3D in a cinema. *ELECTIM.* 2012;21(1):011006-011001-011006-011008.
17. Kooi FL, Toet A. Visual comfort of binocular and 3D displays. *Displays.* 2004;25(2–3):99–108.
18. Javidi B, Okano F. *Three-dimensional television, video, and display technologies.* New York: Springer Science & Business Media; 2002.
19. Huang K, Yuan J-C, Tsai C-H, Hsueh W-J, Wang N-Y. How crosstalk affects stereopsis in stereoscopic displays. *Paper presented at: Electronic Imaging;* 2003.
20. Tam WJ, Speranza F, Yano S, Shimono K, Ono H. Stereoscopic 3D-TV: visual comfort. *IEEE Trans Broadcast.* 2011;57(2):335–346.
21. Yano S, Ide S, Mitsuhashi T, Thwaites H. A study of visual fatigue and visual comfort for 3D HDTV/HDTV images. *Displays.* 2002;23(4):191–201.

22. Li H-CO, Seo J, Kham K, Lee S. Measurement of 3D visual fatigue using event-related potential (ERP): 3D oddball paradigm. *Paper presented at: 2008 3DTV Conference: The True Vision-Capture, Transmission and Display of 3D Video*; 2008.

23. Ujike H, Watanabe H. Effects of stereoscopic presentation on visually induced motion sickness. *Paper presented at: IS&T/SPIE Electronic Imaging*; 2011.

24. IJsselsteijn WA, de Ridder H, Vliegen J. Effects of stereoscopic filming parameters and display duration on the subjective assessment of eye strain. *Paper presented at: Electronic Imaging*; 2000.

25. Cho EJ, Lee KM. Effects of 3D displays: a comparison between shuttered and polarized displays. *Displays.* 2013;34(5):353–358.

26. Malik AS, Khairuddin RNHR, Amin HU, et al. EEG based evaluation of stereoscopic 3D displays for viewer discomfort. *BioMed Eng OnLine.* 2015;14:21.

27. Qi SC, Yan YH, Li R, Hu J. The impact of active versus passive use of 3D technology: a study of dental students at Wuhan University, China. *J Dent Educ.* 2013;77(11):1536–1542.

28. Fehn C, Hopf K, Quante B. Key technologies for an advanced 3D TV system. *Paper presented at: Optics East*; 2004.

29. Goldmann L, De Simone F, Ebrahimi T. A comprehensive database and subjective evaluation methodology for quality of experience in stereoscopic video. *Paper presented at: IS&T/SPIE Electronic Imaging*; 2010.

30. Lambooij M, IJsselsteijn WA, Heynderickx I. Visual discomfort of 3D TV: assessment methods and modeling. *Displays.* 2011;32(4):209–218.

31. Lambooij MT, IJsselsteijn WA, Heynderickx I. Visual discomfort in stereoscopic displays: a review. *Paper presented at: Electronic Imaging*; 2007.

32. Blake R, Wilson H. Binocular vision. *Vision Res.* 2011;51(7):754–770.

33. Kennedy DP, Courchesne E. The intrinsic functional organization of the brain is altered in autism. *Neuroimage.* 2008;39(4):1877–1885.

34. Neri P, Bridge H, Heeger DJ. Stereoscopic processing of absolute and relative disparity in human visual cortex. *J Neurophysiol.* 2004;92(3):1880–1891.

35. Qian N. Binocular disparity and the perception of depth. *Neuron.* 1997;18(3):359–368.

36. Howard IP. Neurons that respond to more than one depth cue. *Trends Neurosci.* 2003;26(10):515–517.

37. Tsao DY, Vanduffel W, Sasaki Y, et al. Stereopsis activates V3A and caudal intraparietal areas in macaques and humans. *Neuron.* 2003;39(3):555–568.

38. Menz MD, Freeman RD. Stereoscopic depth processing in the visual cortex: a coarse-to-fine mechanism. *Nat Neurosci.* 2003;6(1):59–65.

39. Anzai A, Chowdhury SA, DeAngelis GC. Coding of stereoscopic depth information in visual areas V3 and V3A. *J Neurosci Offic J Soc Neurosci.* 2011;31(28):10270–10282.

40. Amin HU, Malik AS, Ahmad RF, et al. Feature extraction and classification for EEG signals using wavelet transform and machine learning techniques. *Australas Phys Eng Sci Med.* 2015;38(1):139–149.

41. Amin HU, Malik AS, Kamel N, Hussain M. A novel approach based on data redundancy for feature extraction of EEG signals. *Brain Topogr.* 2016;29(2):207–217.

42. Amin HU, Malik AS, Subhani AR, Badruddin N, Chooi W-T. Dynamics of scalp potential and autonomic nerve activity during intelligence test. Lee M.Hirose A, Hou Z-G, Kil R, editors. *Neural Information Processing*, Vol 8226. Berlin Heidelberg: Springer; 2013:9–16.

43. Kennedy RS, Lane NE, Berbaum KS, Lilienthal MG. Simulator sickness questionnaire: an enhanced method for quantifying simulator sickness. *Int J Aviat Psychol.* 1993;3(3):203–220.

CHAPTER 7

2D and 3D Educational Contents

Contents

7.1 INTRODUCTION

Three-dimensional (3D) technology has become part of our daily lives with the advent of 3D consumer electronics during the first decade of the 21st century. 3D consumer electronics include all aspects of our digital life including 3D HDTV, 3D DSLR cameras, 3D video cameras, 3D mobile phones, 3D game players, 3D Blu-ray disk players, and 3D PCs. 3D content generation and 3D broadcasting are playing active roles to make 3D technology successful and acceptable for everyday usage. There are many different potential applications of 3D technology, including education, training, and experimentation.[1] With the usage of multimedia educational tools, the teaching and learning process has undergone a revolution since 2000. Sooner or later, 3D multimedia tools will be used in the education sector for academic learning. Hence, in this chapter, we will

Designing EEG Experiments for Studying the Brain.
DOI: http://dx.doi.org/10.1016/B978-0-12-811140-6.00007-2
© 2017 Elsevier Inc.
All rights reserved.

discuss an electroencephalography (EEG) dataset recorded during learning and memorization investigation via 2D and 3D educational contents. EEG signals can capture brain neuronal activities in terms of voltage potentials, which can be analyzed using computational techniques to extract useful information for assessment of brain behavior and activated brain regions.[2,3] In previous studies, EEG has been used for assessment of visual discomfort and fatigue related to 3D displays.[4] The following sections will describe the problem of investigation, software and hardware, experimental design and protocol, and details of EEG data and behavioral data to be used in future by other researchers.

7.2 IMPORTANCE OF STUDYING 3D-BASED MULTIMEDIA EDUCATIONAL TOOLS

The key role of stereoscopic 3D (S3D) based multimedia educational contents in learning complex science concepts and learning new knowledge is obvious from the recent previous studies investigating the impact of S3D multimedia educational content.[5-10] S3D multimedia educational contents play an effective role in understanding complex science concepts, such as medical subjects, by allowing the students to zoom in on the microscopic and cellular levels and rapidly move from watching a complete structure to different parts of the object. One of the first studies of S3D effects on learning and memory retention was reported in 2011 by Anne Bamford.[11] The study reported that S3D helped the students to understand greater levels of complexity and gave them the feeling of reality. The reported results showed that S3D had a significant positive effect on learning, understanding, and memory retention, as well as enhancing the students' engagement, interest, and communication. Overall, 86% of the students had enhanced learning in the S3D class as compared to 52% in the 2D class. In addition, an average of 17% memory retention was improved in the 3D class as compared to only 8% improvement in the 2D class between pretest and posttest of watching the learning content. A recent study reviewed the literature on the comparison of 2D and S3D displays.[12] In this review, 10 studies out of 13 have reported S3D as being better than the 2D display in the understanding of content and memory recall. Price and Lee[13] have investigated the S3D presentation effects on students' performance in cognitive tasks compared to a traditional 2D display. The study reported no difference in response accuracy but a significantly greater task completion time in the S3D presentation. The authors pointed out that the increased number of mental manipulations caused the faster task completion time in the S3D presentation. Korakakis and colleagues[14] investigated S3D versus 2D multimedia contents for science learning and reported that S3D animations enhanced the interest of the students and learning material become more attractive to them.

The findings of these studies are based on subjective feedback of the participants, i.e., either filling out questionnaires or attempting a recall test.[15,16] In such an assessment, it is unknown why and how the physiological effects of S3D-based educational contents help the learners to understand and remember in a better way as compared to traditional 2D contents. Some studies reported the physiological measures, such as pupil size or accommodation responses and eye blinking, for studying the S3D impact on human performances and the visual and/or quality issues.[17–20] But these studies are unable to explain the brain functions, e.g., if the S3D gives good results on various tasks, what is the neuronal mechanism underlying the processing of that information inside the brain, and if the S3D has little to no or effect on human performance in certain tasks, then what is the brain behavior in relation to the tasks where significant differences are not induced?

Recently, some studies employed multimodal assessment including subjective measurements as well as neuroimaging techniques such as EEG for studying S3D.[21,22] However, the problems with these studies are that they focused on the quality issues of S3D, regardless of the neuronal mechanisms being used by the brain cells to process and manipulate the stereoscopic 3D information. Therefore, the underlying brain mechanisms during studying and memory retrieval processes are unclear and need to be investigated using neuroimaging techniques, such as EEG.

The EEG technique is more suitable than any other technique because of its flexibility, cost, and ease of use in experimental environments. EEG enables us to understand the brain neural processes during learning new concepts from S3D contents, which contain disparity and depth information. Hence, the neuronal mechanisms involved in the information processing of S3D contents during learning will explore the reasons for improvement in learning and the overall physiological effects.

7.3 PROBLEM STATEMENT

Research on 2D- and 3D-based educational tools for learning has focused on behavioral feedback, and brain electrophysiological responses are rarely used and in general are neglected.[14,23–33] Similarly, in the memory investigation research, mostly 2D objects are used as stimuli and memory processes are investigated using simple tasks,[34–39] such as learning and recalling words/nouns. However, the use of 3D educational contents along with EEG behavior is not reported. Therefore, the following two research questions were investigated in this experiment and the corresponding dataset:

1. Do students learn, retain, and recall more information when using 3D-based educational tools as compared to traditional 2D tools?
2. Do 3D contents affect short-term and long-term memory (LTM) retention and recall?

All the tasks included in this dataset explore different aspects of human memory including short-term and long-term retention, and the learning process. The purpose and importance of each task are discussed in the experimental design section (Section 7.5).

7.4 SOFTWARE AND HARDWARE

The following software and hardware were used in the collection and organization of this dataset.

1. Electrical Geodesics, Inc. (128-channel EEG equipment with Net Station software)
2. LG stereoscopic TV with 3D polarized glasses (model no. 42LW5700-TA)
3. E-Prime 2.0 (for stimulus experiment design)
4. Autodesk 3D Max 2012 (for making 3DS stimulus)
5. MATLAB 2010 (for simulation)
6. IBM SPSS Statistics 20.0 (Statistical Package for Social Sciences) for data analysis
7. Power Analysis of Sample Size (PASS) for sample size calculation

Autodesk 3DStudioMax: 3DStudioMax (http://www.autodesk.com/) was used for the preparation of 3D objects, which were used as stimuli in working memory and recognition memory tasks. The detail of tasks is provided in the experimental design section (Section 7.5).

E-Prime: E-Prime is psychology software for stimulus presentation in cognitive and behavioral research experiments (http://www.pstnet.com/eprime.cfm). This software allows the users to control time synchronization of stimulus onset, offset, participants' responses, and the corresponding EEG data. All the tasks used during this dataset are explained in the experimental design section (Section 7.5). The details of the E-Prime program for each task are provided in the data description section.

Net Station: Net Station is EEG acquisition software, which was used for recording the EEG signals during the learning and memory tasks. Net Station allows connection with E-Prime software during running the experiments for synchronization of time information of stimulus and participants' responses. The raw EEG recording can be processed in Net Station; its capabilities include filtering, segmentation, rereferencing, and exporting data to several other formats, e.g., .edf or .mat.

EGI 300 Amplifier and EEG nets: The hardware including the EEG nets and amplifier was used from EGI Inc. (http://www.egi.com/). The EEG net used contained 128 channels for recording of dense array EEG from all over the scalp surface locations.

MATLAB: MATLAB is a high-performance programming language for technical computing and coding for engineering problems. It provides an integrative environment to be used by engineers and scientists worldwide. The easy-to-use programming environment of MATLAB provides fast solutions to complex mathematical problems. The well-known disciplines of MATLAB programming are signal and image processing, communications and control systems, computational neuroscience and GUI programming, pattern recognition and machine learning. For beginners in neuroscience, the book *MATLAB for Neuroscientists* by Pascal Wallisch et al. can be consulted.

Statistical Package for Social Sciences: The SPSS was initially designed for social science problems by IBM. However, the software now includes many machine learning algorithms such as clustering and classification. SPSS is widely accepted for statistical analysis including engineering and neuroscience.

Power Analysis of Sample Size: PASS is a software package developed by NCSS, USA. The PASS software provides sample size tools over 680 statistical tests and confidence interval scenarios, validated with published research. The software has become the leading tool for sample size computation in clinical trials, as well as pharmaceutical and other medical research.

7.5 EXPERIMENTAL DESIGN AND PROTOCOL

7.5.1 Target Population

The target population is the possible respondents that may meet the selected set of criteria. All the students on the university campus were the entire set of units for which the findings of the research had been generalized. Three levels of students were studying on the campus at the time of data collection, i.e., foundation level, undergraduate level, and postgraduate level. Equal opportunity to become a participant was provided to all the students who met the inclusion criteria.

7.5.2 Inclusion Criteria

This was the basic set of criteria that must be fulfilled by the student to become a participant in the experiment. It included:

- Participant must be a student in Universiti Teknologi PETRONAS
- Participant should be between 18 and 30 years of age
- Participant must be physically and mentally healthy
- Participant should be available on the campus
- Participant should not have background knowledge in biology

7.5.3 Exclusion Criteria

The exclusion criteria were the requirements that were used for the exclusion of participant from this study. The participants were excluded in this study when they:

- Failed to provide written consent
- Failed to meet the requirements asked in the screening questionnaire

7.5.4 Sample Size Calculation

For comparing means of two independent groups with repeated measure:

- Data types: Outcome variables are numeric (continuous)
- Experiment: Comparison of 3D contents with 2D for memory retention and recall process
- Design: Participants will be randomly assigned into 3D group and 2D group
- Analysis: Two-sample independent t-test at alpha 0.05 (one sided)
      Parameters Specified:
- Power (1-Beta): 80%
- Difference between two means: 0.5 (used Cohen's d for medium sample)
- Standard deviation (assumed to be equal for both groups): 1
- Number of repetitions: 4
- Sample calculated: Group sample sizes of 26 and 26 achieve 80% power to detect a difference of 0.06 in a design with 4 repeated measurements having a compound symmetry covariance structure when the standard deviation was 0.11, and the alpha level is 0.050. Further, keeping 30% margin due to repetition, the total sample size was $N = 68$ (34 for each group)

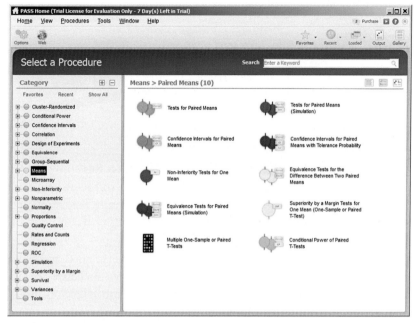

Figure 7.1 PASS user interface window.

- Tool used: We used PASS software (see the main window of PASS in Fig. 7.1) for this calculation. The report is generated by the software with the previously specified parameters.

7.5.5 Participant Recruitment

The study was conducted at University of Technology, PETRONAS. Students from different departments were recruited to participate in the study based on the inclusion criteria. For recruitment, we advertised the invitation for participation in the study on UTP E-learning (http:// elearning.utp.edu.my), and displayed a pamphlet on notice boards in student residential hostels and in cafeterias. Potential participants who responded for participation were recruited based on inclusion criteria and contacted for participation as per their given contact details and asked for to fill out a data collection form.

7.5.6 Experiment Design

In this study, the participants were divided into two groups: one group of participants was tested with 2D contents while another group was tested with 3D contents. Before starting the experiment, participants went through a screening procedure, where they had completed a screening

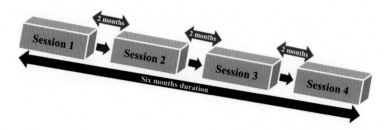

Figure 7.2 Experiment design.

questionnaire and performed an intelligence test. As in this study the participants were called one by one for the experiment, so the assignment of participants to 2D or 3D group had been done randomly (e.g., participant #1 for 2D, participant #2 for 3D, participant #3 for 2D, participant #4 for 3D, and so on).

The experiment consisted of four sessions; experimental tasks were distributed among the sessions. The gap between two successive sessions was 8 weeks/2 months. This 2-month interval was the retention interval (see Fig. 7.2).

The following is the list of the experimental tasks used in the study:
• general cognitive ability task (Session 1)
• learning task (Sessions 1, 2, and 3)
• oddball task (Session 1)
• memory recall task (Sessions 1, 2, 3, and 4)

7.5.6.1 General Cognitive Ability Task

Raven's Advanced Progressive Matrices (RAPM) is used to measure high-level observation skills, thinking ability, intellectual efficiency, and intellectual capacity. This RAPM kit was purchased from the Western Psychology Society and it was developed by Pearson Education Inc. It is administered as per instructions provided with the kit by the publisher. The raw score of this test indicated the participants' ability to make sense of complex situations. It consisted of 12 items for the practice session and 36 items for the test session and the recommended time duration was 30–40 minutes. Each item was a pattern with a missing element and four possible options. Only one option was the correct part of the pattern to be selected. A sample RAPM problem is provided in Fig. 7.3 (the correct answer in this case is 7). This task was performed by every participant of each group in the first session of the experiment. The raw score was used to control the nonexperimental variable "intelligence" in both groups.

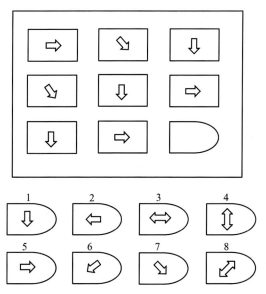

Figure 7.3 A sample of Raven's Advanced Progressive Matrices (RAPM) problem.[40]

7.5.6.2 Learning Task (3D Animation)

For learning and memory retention purposes, this task consisted of 3D stereoscopic animations of the biology course. To avoid participants with background knowledge regarding the animations, participants were recruited having no or very little knowledge of biology. Thus, the participants would find the biology animations to be new knowledge and during watching the content, new memory traces would be formed. In this task, three animations were shown and each animation was repeated three times. The duration of the animated contents was approximately 10 minutes and it was repeated three times; hence, approximately 30 minutes were spent in the learning task. This task was used in the first three sessions. However, in the second and third sessions, the learning contents were presented once, i.e., for 10 minutes only.

7.5.6.3 Visual Oddball Task

The purpose of this task was to check if there were any aftereffects of 3D viewing in terms of mental fatigue and/or visual discomfort. In case a participant was fatigued due to 3D viewing, the amplitude of P300 would be suppressed.[41,42] The details and experimental data of this task will be discussed in Chapter 8, Visual and Cognitive Fatigue During Learning, of this book.

Q. The damage of epithelial wall activates the platelets to form_____.

1. Fibrin thread

2. Good cholesterol

3. HDL

4. Clot

Figure 7.4 Sample of multiple choice question (MCQ).[40]

7.5.6.4 Recall Task

A recall task was presented that was composed of 20 multiple choice questions (MCQs) about all three animations that the participants studied during the learning task. The recall task was conducted 30 minutes after the learning task for short-term memory recall. Then in second session, after a duration of 2 months (8 weeks), the recall task was performed to check for LTM recall. This was repeated in sessions 3 and 4. An example MCQ is provided in Fig. 7.4.

7.5.7 Experiment Procedure

This experiment consisted of four sessions (see Fig. 7.5). In the first session, when a participant arrived at the experiment room, he/she was informed of the experiment (see Appendix 14) and asked to sign a consent form (see Appendix 2C). Participants provided consent, completed a screening questionnaire containing questions related to medical history, medications, and demographics (Appendix 7A), and performed an RAPM test to control for intelligence. Following the screening procedure, a compatible EEG electrode cap was put on the participant's head, and then EEG data were recorded at rest state (eyes-closed and eyes-open conditions).

After the baseline EEG recording, the participant was exposed to the animated contents either in 3D mode or 2D mode depending upon the participant's group. The participant watched and learned information provided in the animated contents and retained the information. Immediately, after the learning task, participant was exposed to the oddball task, which lasted approximately 4 minutes. A 30-minute retention time was given to participants including the duration of oddball task. After the retention time, the participant performed the memory recall task. Then EEG electrode cap was removed and the participant completed a feedback questionnaire containing questions related to learning environment (2D or 3D), participant's perception, and experiment procedure (Appendix 7B). At the end of this

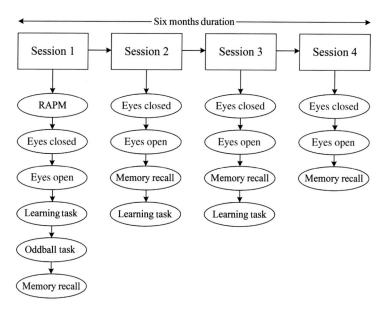

Figure 7.5 Experimental design with session wise tasks.

first session, the participant was requested to participate for a second session (after two months) for a memory recall task to determine LTM retention and rehearsal of the contents (2D/3D animation).

In the second session, an EEG electrode cap was put on the participant's head, and EEG data was recorded at rest state (eyes-closed, eyes-open conditions). Next, the participant performed a memory recall task in which the participant had to recall the 2D or 3D contents learned in the first session. EEG data was recorded during the recall task. After the recall test, the participant watched the same animated contents (learning task) again for rehearsal. At the end of the second session, the participant was reminded to come for the third session after two months for the same retrieval task. The same procedure of session 2 was repeated in the third and fourth sessions. However, in the fourth session, the animated contents (learning task) were not presented again, as it was the last session.

7.6 DATA DESCRIPTION

The details of the EEG data from session 1 are described in Table 7.1.

The details of tasks for sessions 2, 3, and 4 are similar except that in session 4 the learning task is not used. The details of the tasks are given in Table 7.2.

Table 7.1 Detail of first session tasks

S. No.	Task	Duration	EEG	Purpose
01	RAPM (general cognitive ability task)	Max. 48 min	No	To control the IQ between the groups
5-min break				
02	Eyes closed	5 min	Yes	Baseline (rest condition)
	Eyes open	5 min	Yes	Baseline (rest condition)
5-min break				
03	Learning task (3D/2D animated contents) The contents were presented total three times	up to 10 min (3 × 10 = 30 minutes)	Yes	Learning a memorization information (Rehearsal for better encoding)
Retention time 30 min between learning task and memory recall task				
04	Oddball task	3.35 min	Yes	Attention and P300
05	Recall task (after 30 min)	Max. 10 min	Yes	Short-term recall in 2D/3D after 30 minutes

Table 7.2 Detail of sessions 2, 3, and 4 tasks

S. No.	Task	Duration	EEG	Purpose
01	Eyes closed	5 min	Yes	Baseline (rest condition)
	Eyes open	5 min	Yes	Baseline (rest condition)
02	Recall task (after 30 min)	Max. 10 min	Yes	Long-term recall in 2D/3D after 2 months
03	Learning task (★This task is not used in session 4)	up to 10 min	Yes	Rehearsing for better encoding

7.6.1 E-Prime Program

The E-Prime programs for the tasks mentioned in Table 7.1 are provided with this book. The tasks are designed using E-Prime version 2.0. The programs are editable and easy to modify. Help on E-Prime is available from the E-Prime manuals available at (step.psy.cmu.edu/materials/manuals).

The E-Prime software package constitutes five programs: E-Studio, E-Run, E-DataAid, E-Merge, and E-Recovery. The E-Studio program is dedicated to creating the experiments (Tasks). The main interface of E-Studio can be seen in Fig. 7.6. It contains structure, ToolBox, Properties, and Worksheet. The details of each of these components are explained in the

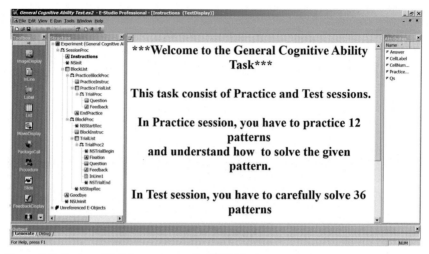

Figure 7.6 Design of E-Prime program for RAPM task.

E-Prime technical manuals. There are a few main building blocks of designing experimental tasks in E-Prime, i.e., frames, blocks, and trials. A frame can be either a slide with text instructions or pictures shown to the participant. The instructions (frame) for the RAPM task are shown in Fig. 7.6, enclosed in a red rectangle. Trials consist of an organization of frames in which the stimuli are presented. The block is a group of trials that contains all necessary frames, from the instruction frame to the conclusion frame.

Let's look at the design of task number 01 (RAPM) in Table 7.1. There are two blocks called "PracticeBlockProc" and "BlockProc." The "PracticeBlockProc" contains 12 trials that were used for practice before going to the actual Raven's test. Each trial consists of a stimulus frame (picture of the problem to be solved) and feedback frame that tells the participant about the correct/incorrect attempt, score, and time taken by the participant to press a button as a response. Similarly, the block "BlockProc" contains 36 trials for the actual experiment. Each trial contains a fixation frame that simply tells the participant that it follows a stimulus frame. The stimulus frame presents a picture of a problem to be solved for assessment of the participant's general cognitive ability. The participant needs to record his/her response by pressing a button as instructed in the instruction frame. After pressing a button, the feedback frame shows the result of the response either as correct or incorrect. There is a frame called "InLine1," which contains a few lines of code to stamp the EEG recording with desired events such as stimulus onset, participants' response, etc.

E-Prime allows recording of all related information in the experiment including stimulus information (stimulus onset, offset, duration etc.),

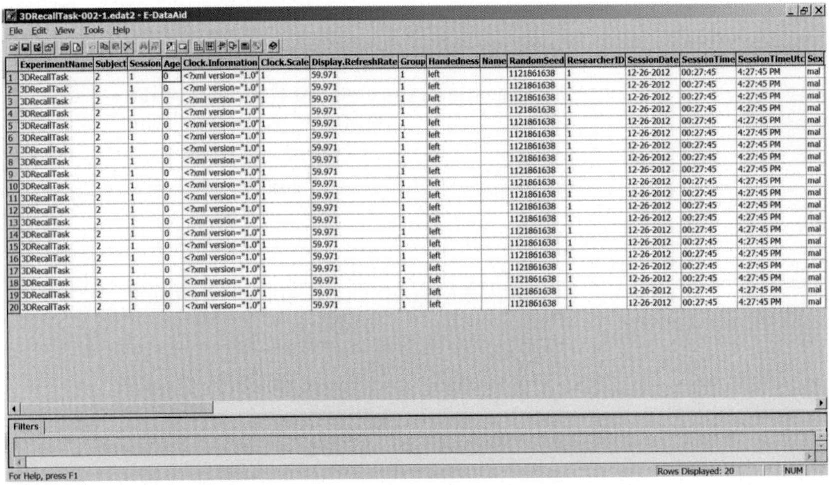

	ExperimentName	Subject	Session	Age	Clock.Information	Clock.Scale	Display.RefreshRate	Group	Handedness	Name	RandomSeed	ResearcherID	SessionDate	SessionTime	SessionTimeUtc	Sex
1	3DRecallTask	2	1	0	<?xml version="1.0"	1	59.971	1	left		1121861638	1	12-26-2012	00:27:45	4:27:45 PM	mal
2	3DRecallTask	2	1	0	<?xml version="1.0"	1	59.971	1	left		1121861638	1	12-26-2012	00:27:45	4:27:45 PM	mal
3	3DRecallTask	2	1	0	<?xml version="1.0"	1	59.971	1	left		1121861638	1	12-26-2012	00:27:45	4:27:45 PM	mal
4	3DRecallTask	2	1	0	<?xml version="1.0"	1	59.971	1	left		1121861638	1	12-26-2012	00:27:45	4:27:45 PM	mal
5	3DRecallTask	2	1	0	<?xml version="1.0"	1	59.971	1	left		1121861638	1	12-26-2012	00:27:45	4:27:45 PM	mal
6	3DRecallTask	2	1	0	<?xml version="1.0"	1	59.971	1	left		1121861638	1	12-26-2012	00:27:45	4:27:45 PM	mal
7	3DRecallTask	2	1	0	<?xml version="1.0"	1	59.971	1	left		1121861638	1	12-26-2012	00:27:45	4:27:45 PM	mal
8	3DRecallTask	2	1	0	<?xml version="1.0"	1	59.971	1	left		1121861638	1	12-26-2012	00:27:45	4:27:45 PM	mal
9	3DRecallTask	2	1	0	<?xml version="1.0"	1	59.971	1	left		1121861638	1	12-26-2012	00:27:45	4:27:45 PM	mal
10	3DRecallTask	2	1	0	<?xml version="1.0"	1	59.971	1	left		1121861638	1	12-26-2012	00:27:45	4:27:45 PM	mal
11	3DRecallTask	2	1	0	<?xml version="1.0"	1	59.971	1	left		1121861638	1	12-26-2012	00:27:45	4:27:45 PM	mal
12	3DRecallTask	2	1	0	<?xml version="1.0"	1	59.971	1	left		1121861638	1	12-26-2012	00:27:45	4:27:45 PM	mal
13	3DRecallTask	2	1	0	<?xml version="1.0"	1	59.971	1	left		1121861638	1	12-26-2012	00:27:45	4:27:45 PM	mal
14	3DRecallTask	2	1	0	<?xml version="1.0"	1	59.971	1	left		1121861638	1	12-26-2012	00:27:45	4:27:45 PM	mal
15	3DRecallTask	2	1	0	<?xml version="1.0"	1	59.971	1	left		1121861638	1	12-26-2012	00:27:45	4:27:45 PM	mal
16	3DRecallTask	2	1	0	<?xml version="1.0"	1	59.971	1	left		1121861638	1	12-26-2012	00:27:45	4:27:45 PM	mal
17	3DRecallTask	2	1	0	<?xml version="1.0"	1	59.971	1	left		1121861638	1	12-26-2012	00:27:45	4:27:45 PM	mal
18	3DRecallTask	2	1	0	<?xml version="1.0"	1	59.971	1	left		1121861638	1	12-26-2012	00:27:45	4:27:45 PM	mal
19	3DRecallTask	2	1	0	<?xml version="1.0"	1	59.971	1	left		1121861638	1	12-26-2012	00:27:45	4:27:45 PM	mal
20	3DRecallTask	2	1	0	<?xml version="1.0"	1	59.971	1	left		1121861638	1	12-26-2012	00:27:45	4:27:45 PM	mal

Figure 7.7 E-Prime recorded file in 3D recall task.

trials information (fixation, intertrials duration, and feedback display), participant responses (reaction time, true and false responses), and recording additional information about the participant or experiment such as participant number, age, gender, handedness, name, session number, group number, date of experiment, start, and end time of session. The print screen of a recorded E-Prime file is shown in Fig. 7.7.

E-Prime also provides an analysis tool to extract the required information from all the files recorded in a particular experiment for individual participant analysis as well as group analysis. The guidelines on how to use the analysis tool of E-Prime for data analysis are mentioned in the manuals, which are available at step.psy.cmu.edu/materials/manuals.

7.6.2 EEG Description

The EEG was recorded via 128 scalp loci using the EGI HydroCel Geodesic Sensor Net with Amps 300 amplifier (Electrical Geodesic Inc., Eugene, OR, USA) for all the tasks. The electrode Cz is used as a reference to all the 128 electrodes. Impedance was maintained below 50 KΩ as per EGI equipment guidelines and the sampling rate was 250 samples/second.

7.6.3 Experiment Data Accompanying this Book

The experimental tasks designed in E-Prime are provided in Table 7.3. EEG raw data, clean data, ERP nonaveraged data, and event files for one participant are provided with this book. The details of these files are provided in Tables 7.4 and 7.5. To access these files, please go to the directory

Table 7.3 E-Prime experiment design files

S. No.	Directory name	Description
01	EC and EO	This directory contains the two E-Prime files for resting state EEG used in all four sessions: (1) EP-NS-EC-01.es2, which is used to start and stop EEG recording for the eyes-closed condition; and (2) EP-NS-EO-01.es2, which is used for the eyes-open condition EEG recording. The function of these experimental files is simple. EP-NS-EC-01.es2 only starts and stops EEG recording automatically during experimentation of the eyes-closed EEG condition. The experimenter does not need to start or stop the EEG recording manually. Similarly, the function of EP-NS-EO-01.es2 is to show a fixation point on the screen along with starting and stopping the EEG recordings.
02	Visual oddball task	This directory contains the visual oddball experiment developed in E-Prime. The details of this visual oddball task are discussed in Chapter 8, Visual and Cognitive Fatigue During Learning.
03	Memory recall task	This directory contains the memory recall task used in all four sessions of the experiment.

Table 7.4 EEG data description of session 1

S. No.	File name	Description
01	EC.mat	Resting state EEG recording for eyes-closed condition.
02	EO.mat	Resting state EEG recording for eyes-open condition.
03	L1.mat	EEG recording during study session. In this recording the participants watched animated learning contents while EEG data was recorded.
04	L2.mat	In the EEG recording, the same animated contents (as shown in S. No. 3) were repeated to better memorize the learning material while EEG was recorded.
05	L3.mat	In the EEG recording, the same animated contents (as shown in S. No. 3) were repeated again to better memorize the learning material while EEG was recorded.
06	S1_Oddball.mat S1_Oddball.evt	This file contains EEG data recorded during presentation of the oddball task. The oddball task is a time-locked event-related potential (ERP) task and contains visual stimuli events. Therefore, the ERP signal can be extracted from this EEG file with the support of the .evt file.
07	S1_recall.mat S1_recall.evt	This file contains EEG data recorded during the memory recall task. This file contains 20 events of question onset and participant response. The .evt file contains the events to be used for analysis of individual questions in each participant or extracting the onset of questions and response time of the participants.

Table 7.5 EEG data description of sessions 2, 3, and 4

S. No.	Session 2	Session 3	Session 4
1	S1_EC.mat	S1_EC.mat	S1_EC.mat
2	S1_EO.mat	S1_EO.mat	S1_EO.mat
3	S1_Recall.mat	S1_Recall.mat	S1_Recall.mat
	S1_Recall.evt	S1_Recall.evt	S1_Recall.evt
4	S1_Learning.mat	x	x

BookData\Chap07\EEG in the data files accompanying this book. The clean and raw EEG data are placed in separate directories. For the complete dataset of 68 participants, please contact the authors at brainexpbook@gmail.com.

7.7 RELEVANT PAPERS

This section provides a list of some of the papers that have utilized the data acquired from the experiment described in this chapter. The following papers should be cited when using the experiment design or the data provided with this chapter.

1. Amin HU, Malik AS, Kamel N, Chooi W-T, Hussain M. P300 correlates with learning & memory abilities and fluid intelligence. *J NeuroEng Rehabil.* 2015;12:1–14.
2. Amin HU, Malik AS, Kamel N, Hussain M. A novel approach based on data redundancy for feature extraction of EEG signals. *Brain Topogr. 2016*; 29:207–217.
3. Amin HU, Malik AS, Mumtaz W, Badruddin N, Kamel N. Evaluation of passive polarized stereoscopic 3D display for visual & mental fatigues. In: *Engineering in Medicine and Biology Society (EMBC), 2015 37th Annual International Conference of the IEEE*; 2015, pp. 7590–7593.

ACKNOWLEDGMENTS

This chapter provides the details of the experiment design available in the papers mentioned in Section 7.7 and in the PhD thesis of Hafeez Ullah Amin, which is available at Universiti Teknologi PETRONAS.

REFERENCES

1. Salmon G. The future for (second) life and learning. *Br J Educ Technol.* 2009;40(3):526–538.
2. Amin HU, Malik AS, Ahmad RF, et al. Feature extraction and classification for EEG signals using wavelet transform and machine learning techniques. *Australas Phys Eng Sci Med.* 2015;38(1):139–149.

3. Amin HU, Malik AS, Kamel N, Hussain M. A novel approach based on data redundancy for feature extraction of EEG signals. *Brain Topogr.* 2016;29(2):207–217.
4. Malik AS, Khairuddin RNHR, Amin HU, et al. EEG based evaluation of stereoscopic 3D displays for viewer discomfort. *BioMed Eng Online.* 2015;14(1):21.
5. Hoyek N, Collet C, Rienzo F, Almeida M, Guillot A. Effectiveness of three-dimensional digital animation in teaching human anatomy in an authentic classroom context. *Anat Sci Educ.* 2014;7(6):430–437.
6. Guillot A, Champely S, Batier C, Thiriet P, Collet C. Relationship between spatial abilities, mental rotation and functional anatomy learning. *Adv Health Sci Educ.* 2007;12(4):491–507.
7. Hegarty M, Keehner M, Cohen C, Montello DR, Lippa Y. The role of spatial cognition in medicine: applications for selecting and training professionals. *Appl Spatial Cognit.* 2007:285–315.
8. Roach VA, Brandt MG, Moore CC, Wilson TD. Is three-dimensional videography the cutting edge of surgical skill acquisition? *Anat Sci Educ.* 2012;5(3):138–145.
9. Malik AS, Amin HU, Badruddin N, Kamel N, Ahmad RF, Mumtaz W. Evaluation of stereoscopic 3D based educational contents for long-term memorization. *Ann Neurol.* 2015;78(S19):S89–S89.
10. Malik AS, Amin HU, Kamel N, Chooi W-T, Hussain M. The effects of 3D technology on the brain during learning and memory recall processes. *Ann Neurol.* 2014;76:S24–S24.
11. Bamford A. The 3D in Education White Paper International Research Agency; 2011.
12. McIntire JP, Havig PR, Geiselman EE. Stereoscopic 3D displays and human performance: a comprehensive review. *Displays.* 2014;35(1):18–26.
13. Price A, Lee H-S. The effect of two-dimensional and stereoscopic presentation on middle school students' performance of spatial cognition tasks. *J Sci Educ Technol.* 2010;19(1):90–103.
14. Korakakis G, Pavlatou EA, Palyvos JA, Spyrellis N. 3D visualization types in multimedia applications for science learning: a case study for 8th grade students in Greece. *Comput Educ.* 2009;52(2):390–401.
15. Kuze J, Ukai K. Subjective evaluation of visual fatigue caused by motion images. *Displays.* 2008;29(2):159–166.
16. Moorthy AK, Su C-C, Mittal A, Bovik AC. Subjective evaluation of stereoscopic image quality. *Signal Process Image Commun.* 2013;28(8):870–883.
17. Takaki Y, Yokouchi M. Accommodation measurements of horizontally scanning holographic display. *Optics Express.* 2012;20(4):3918–3931.
18. Wang D, Wang T, Gong Y. Stereoscopic visual fatigue assessment and modeling. *Paper presented at: IS&T/SPIE Electronic Imaging;* 2014.
19. Kim D, Choi S, Park S, Sohn K. Stereoscopic visual fatigue measurement based on fusional response curve and eye-blinks. *Paper presented at: 2011 17th International Conference on Digital Signal Processing (DSP);* 2011.
20. Iatsun I, Larabi M-C, Fernandez-Maloigne C. Investigation and modeling of visual fatigue caused by S3D content using eye-tracking. *Displays.* 2015;39:11–25.
21. Chen C, Li K, Wu Q, Wang H, Qian Z, Sudlow G. EEG-based detection and evaluation of fatigue caused by watching 3DTV. *Displays.* 2013;34(2):81–88.
22. Chen C, Wang J, Li K, et al. Assessment visual fatigue of watching 3DTV using EEG power spectral parameters. *Displays.* 2014;35(5):266–272.
23. Ciobanu O, Tornincasa S. The use of dynamic interactive 3D images of biomedical devices in education. *Paper Presented at: Second International Conference in Visualization,* Barcelona; 2009.
24. Iqbal T, Hammermüller K, Tjoa AM. *Second life for illiterates: a 3D virtual world platform for Adult Basic Education,* Paris; 2010.
25. Settapat S, Achalakul T, Ohkura M. Web-based 3D medical image visualization framework for biomedical engineering education. *Comput Appl Eng Educ.* 2014;22(2):216–226.

26. Kamsin A, Cha Gek T, Tay Lee K. The Implementation of a Web-based 3D Multimedia Learning Prototype in Biology subject: BioID. *Paper presented at: Innovations in Information Technology, 2007. IIT '07. 4th International Conference; November 18–20, 2007.*

27. Kamsin A, Abdullah MYH. The development of 3D Multimedia Learning Tool (MLTBS) in Information Communication Technology (ICT) for teaching and learning purposes. *Paper presented at: Proceedings of the International Conference on Computer Graphics, Imaging and Visualisation (CGIV'06),* Sydney; 2006.

28. Perez FL, Vanegas SIC, Cortes PEC. Evaluation of learning processes applying 3D models for constructive processes from solutions to problems. *Paper presented at: Education Technology and Computer (ICETC), 2010, 2nd International Conference;* June 22–24, 2010.

29. Ranky PG. *Interactive 3D multimedia cases for engineering education with internet support,* Nashville, TN; 2003.

30. Ranky PG. A *novel 3D Internet-based multimedia method for teaching and learning about engineering management requirements analysis,* Nashville, TN; 2003.

31. Borissova D, Mustakerov I. A framework of multimedia E-learning design for engineering. Spaniol M. Li Q, Klamma R, Lau R, editors. *Training Advances in Web Based Learning–ICWL 2009,* Vol 5686. Berlin/Heidelberg: Springer; 2009:88–97.

32. Brenton H, Hernandez J, Bello F, et al. Using multimedia and Web3D to enhance anatomy teaching. *Comput Educ.* 2007;49(1):32–53.

33. Moos DC, Marroquin E. Multimedia, hypermedia, and hypertext: motivation considered and reconsidered. *Comput Human Behav.* 2010;26(3):265–276.

34. Karlsgodt KH, Shirinyan D, van Erp TG, Cohen MS, Cannon TD. Hippocampal activations during encoding and retrieval in a verbal working memory paradigm. *Neuroimage.* 2005;25(4):1224–1231.

35. Banko EM, Vidnyanszky Z. Retention interval affects visual short-term memory encoding. *J. Neurophysiol.* 2010;103(3):1425–1430.

36. Joiner WM, Smith MA. Long-term retention explained by a model of short-term learning in the adaptive control of reaching. *J Neurophysiol.* 2008;100(5):2948–2955.

37. Babiloni C, Babiloni F, Carducci F, et al. Human cortical EEG rhythms during long-term episodic memory task. A high-resolution EEG study of the HERA model. *Neuroimage.* 2004;21(4):1576–1584.

38. Burgess AP, Gruzelier JH. Short duration power changes in the EEG during recognition memory for words and faces. *Psychophysiology.* 2000;37(5):596–606.

39. Chen Xue-li YB, Dong-yu WU, et al. Application of EEG non-linear analysis in vision memory study. *Chin J Rehabil Theory Pract.* 2006.

40. Amin HU, Malik AS, Kamel N, Chooi W-T, Hussain M. P300 correlates with learning & memory abilities and fluid intelligence. *J NeuroEng Rehabil.* 2015;12(1):87.

41. Amin HU, Malik AS, Mumtaz W, Badruddin N, Kamel N. Evaluation of passive polarized stereoscopic 3D display for visual & mental fatigues. *Paper presented at: Engineering in Medicine and Biology Society (EMBC), 2015 37th Annual International Conference of the IEEE; August 25–29, 2015.*

42. Amin HU, Malik AS, Badruddin N, Kamel N, Hussain M. Effects of stereoscopic 3D display technology on event-related potentials (ERPs). *Paper presented at: Neural Engineering (NER), 2015 7th International IEEE/EMBS Conference;* April 22–24, 2015.

CHAPTER 8

Visual and Cognitive Fatigue During Learning

Contents

8.1 INTRODUCTION

Today, in the entertainment market, stereoscopic three-dimensional (S3D) technologies have been growing rapidly, especially for the two commonly used 3D display technologies—active shutter and passive polarized. Active shuttered 3D creates the illusion of a 3D image by using active shuttered glasses and showing the images alternatively in a sequential manner to each eye in synchronization with the refresh rate of the screen. Active shuttered glasses contain liquid crystal and a polarizing filter alternately blocks one eye lens and then the other when voltage is applied.[1] Passive polarized 3D projects each image with mutually orthogonal polarizations and each eye perceives a different image simultaneously due to polarizing glasses.

Despite the rapid and growing developments in 3D technology, 3D visual discomfort, visual fatigue, and mental fatigue continue to be reported.[2,3] The visual discomfort is a perceived degree of annoyance assessed by the viewers themselves during watching S3D contents or any negative sensation related to a given visual task.[2] It can be measured by simply asking the viewers to report their experience of watching S3D

Designing EEG Experiments for Studying the Brain.
DOI: http://dx.doi.org/10.1016/B978-0-12-811140-6.00008-4
© 2017 Elsevier Inc.
All rights reserved.
123

contents. However, it may appear and disappear rapidly by viewers closing their eyes, diverting their focus from the screen, or terminating the visual task. In contrast, visual fatigue and mental fatigue are supposed to have longer rise and fall time than visual discomfort. The presence of visual and mental fatigues may be evaluated with a subjective method, i.e., one or several symptoms reported by the viewers (e.g., nausea) and also by objective measurement such as eye blinking rate[4,5] and event-related potentials (ERPs).[3,6] In addition, the visual and mental fatigue continues for some time even after the S3D viewing is finished. It may not be diagnosed instantly in conjunction with a certain S3D-based visual task.[2]

In this experiment, S3D-based educational contents were assessed for mental fatigue during the learning process using electrophysiological signals (EEG/ERP and ECG). EEG/ERP signals are well known for measuring neuronal changes during any task. The association of dynamics in ECG signals with EEG signals during the cognitive process is reported using heart rate variability (HRV) analysis.[7] This experiment is a part of Chapter 7, 2D and 3D Educational Contents, in which S3D effects were explored for memory retention. However, the experiment part that will be discussed in this chapter is focused on another research objective, i.e., mental fatigue assessment during the learning process for S3D-based educational contents. The experimental design and physiological data acquisition will be discussed in this chapter in Section 8.4.

8.2 IMPORTANCE AND SIGNIFICANCE OF VISUAL AND MENTAL FATIGUE DURING LEARNING

In S3D research, quality aspects with respect to the satisfaction of the viewers are widely studied.[8,9] The viewers' complaints and feedback have been recorded in many experiments for further improvement in S3D quality.[10,11] The most commonly investigated quality factors are 3D cross talk,[12] comfort/discomfort,[8,13] cognitive and visual fatigue,[14,15] motion sickness,[16] aftereffects,[17] and 3D effects on vision.[18] This visual and mental fatigue from S3D vision in entertainment such as watching movies or playing games may not be so serious because the viewers are entertaining themselves rather using S3D for serious purposes such as education. However, the appearance of such visual or mental fatigue during the learning process cannot be ignored.[19,20] In the learning process, if the learners feel visual strain and/or heavy head due to watching the S3D content, their focus and concentration will be lost. Thus, it will cause distraction to the attentional resources that are necessary for perceiving new knowledge.

Visual fatigue and discomfort are not only issues with S3D but also occur with extensive use of computer screens or any visual display, such as TV. It has been investigated that the excessive use of display screens may cause eye strain, headache, visual discomfort, fatigue, and other negative effects.[21,22] The reason for these symptoms with normal visual display is the screen low refresh rate. If the refresh rate is too low, it will cause screen flickering. Thus the flashing of light may induce negative effects, such as photosensitive seizures.[23] It has been reported that an individual may experience motion sickness in front of a large visual display,[24] which may be due to rapid eye movements.

In case of S3D, the symptoms of visual discomfort and fatigue are studied using subjective and/or physiological measures.[2,10,13,25–27] It is one of the most frequent complaints of S3D viewers and considered an important dimension of the quality of experience of S3D. The reason for this widely studied factor is obvious as it concerns the health and safety of the viewers.[2] Visual discomfort is the perception of the degree of annoyance during performing a visual task and can be measured as suggested by Li et al.[2], to ask the viewers to report his/her experience. However, visual discomfort may disappear quickly if the participant is distracted or closes his/her eyes. In addition, visual fatigue is differentiated by Lambooij[27] from visual discomfort, i.e., visual fatigue is the decrease in performance of visual system due to the physiological changes. Therefore, it can be measured with EEG or ERPs, which are physiological measures and reflect the neuronal mechanisms directly.

8.3 PROBLEM STATEMENT

Many studies had used subjective and objectives methods for measurements of visual and mental fatigue, such as questionnaire-based subjective assessment, pupil tracking and eye blinking rate, and biosignals–based objective evaluation.[3–5,28] ERPs are an objective measurement method of visual and mental fatigue, which directly reflect the cognitive state of the brain.[28] The P300 (P3) component is strongly associated to the level of attention and reflects the degree of stimulus processing cognitively.[29] It has been shown that the P3 amplitude provoked by cognitive task loading decreases due to an increase in the cognitive task difficulty.[29] Therefore, it is useful to assess the depth of cognitive information processing. The visual and mental fatigue induced by cognitive loading due to watching S3D videos can be measured by the ERP components, i.e., decreased P3 amplitude and prolonged P3 latency reveal that visual and mental fatigue are induced.[28,30,31]

However, the previous studies reported visual and mental fatigue for active shuttered 3D display.[30,32] Thus, an important question arises as to whether the passive polarized S3D display also induces such effects (visual and mental fatigue) as reported for the active shuttered 3D display. In addition, the previous studies used ERPs as objective measurement for visual and mental fatigue but did not consider the intelligence ability of the participants, which is correlated with the ERP components, e.g., high P3 amplitude at the centroparietal regions is positively correlated with individuals' intelligence ability.[33] Thus, if two separate groups of participants are exposed to 2D and S3D contents then their intelligence ability may be a factor of biasness if it is not controlled. Moreover, the previous studies did not use stereoscopic 3D visual stimuli in the ERP tasks. They used 2D-based visual stimuli in the oddball task.[31,34] It is obvious that visual or mental fatigue often disappears after some time of 3D visualization. Therefore, in this study the visual stimuli in the oddball task were 3D based for the S3D group and 2D-based for the 2D group. Thus, if fatigue occurred in the S3D group due to S3D visualization, it should not disappear in the ERP recording. This study evaluated visual and mental fatigue using ERP for passive polarized S3D display and compared with traditional 2D display by employing a sample of 68 healthy participants. The participants are equally categorized into 2D and S3D groups, while their age and fluid intelligence ability are tightly controlled between groups.

Besides the P300 component, it was reported in previous studies that autonomic nervous activities (HRV) are affected due to watching 3D films. Chen et al.[35] reported that parasympathetic nerve activities were reduced after visualization of 3D movies and concluded that this may be a sign of tiredness, discomfort, and fatigue as reflected by participants' complaints recorded in the questionnaire filled out after watching movies. Park et al.[32] reported that autonomic balance and heart rhythm change due to viewing stereoscopic 3D contents. In their results, a significant increase in heart rate (HR) was observed in the 3D group that reflected arousal and an increase in very low frequency/high frequency ratio (VLF/HF) was also reported in the 3D group compared to the 2D group, which indicated that autonomic balance was not stable. They concluded that 3D viewing induces lasting activation in the sympathetic nervous system and an interruption in autonomic balance. These studies have used movie contents and the display technology was active shutter 3D. However, the S3D-based educational content may or may not induce such effects with passive polarized 3D display.

On the basis of technological differences between active shuttered and passive polarized displays and considering the related studies investigating the visual and mental fatigue of active shuttered 3D display,[30,32] it was hypothesized in this research that the amplitude of P3 of the S3D group would be reduced if visual and/or mental fatigue occurs as compared to the 2D group.[36] The basis of the hypothesis is that relatively fewer attentional resources are available when an individual is in a cognitive fatigue state, which resists focusing and divides attention between visual stimuli.[34] Thus, that affects the P3 amplitude and latency. Furthermore, the P200 (P2) of ERP is associated with the secondary processing of visual input and is partially involved in cognitive processing.[37] Therefore, the P2 component was included in the analysis. In addition, the HRV would be increased if the viewers experienced discomfort and mental fatigue.

8.4 SOFTWARE AND HARDWARE

In this experiment, the software and hardware utilization was almost the same as in the experiment tasks discussed in Chapter 7, 2D and 3D Educational Contents. However, the additional equipment adopted for the recording of ECG signals is described here.

1. EGI Polygraph Input Box (PIB): The PIB is physiological measurement system provided by EGI. It is capable of recording the peripheral nervous system activity and EEG signals simultaneously. The PIB consists of seven bipolar channel inputs for measurement of ECG, EMG (electromyogram), respiration (temperature and pressure), and body position (see Fig. 8.1). The PIB does not require any separate software setup and is embedded in Net Station 4.4 or later version. The Net Station software (as explained in Chapter 7, 2D and 3D Educational Contents) consists of a toggle button on the toolbar that shows or hides all the PIB channels.

2. Biosignal Toolbox: This is an open source software library for biomedical signal processing available for both MATLAB and C++ platforms for data analysis. The source code can be downloaded from http://biosig.sourceforge.net/download.html. The applications of this toolbox include analysis of electroencephalogram (EEG), electrocorticogram (ECoG), electrocardiogram (ECG), electrooculogram (EOG), EMG, and respiration data.

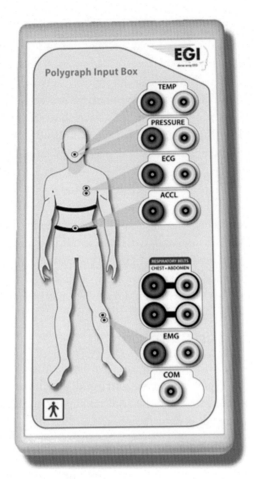

Figure 8.1 Polygraphic Input Box (PIB).

8.5 EXPERIMENT DESIGN AND PROTOCOL

This chapter is a part of the experiment described in Chapter 7, 2D and 3D Educational Contents. Thus, the details of target population, inclusion criteria, exclusion criteria, sample size computation, and participants have already been provided in Chapter 7, 2D and 3D Educational Contents. Here, the experimental design tasks and the procedure, which are not covered in the previous chapter, are described.

8.5.1 Experiment Design

In this study, the participants were divided into two groups: one group of participants was tested with 2D learning contents while another group was tested with 3D learning contents. As mentioned in Chapter 7, 2D and 3D Educational Contents, the individual participants' reasoning and general cognitive ability were assessed using Raven's Advanced Progressive Matrices (RAPM) test. The RAPM task was also required while analyzing the ERP components for mental fatigue. The reason is that the relationship of ERP components and general intelligence is reported in previous studies. Hence, the RAPM data of the participants was also required in this chapter along with the learning task (watching learning animated contents with 3D or 2D display) and oddball tasks for ERP signal analysis. The RAPM and learning task is briefly touched on here, and the oddball task is described in detail.

The following is the list of the experimental tasks used in the study:
- Raven's Advanced Progressive Matrices (RAPM) test
- 3D visualization
- oddball task

8.5.1.1 Raven's Advanced Progressive Matrices (RAPM) Test

RAPM test is a nonverbal standard psychometric test used to measure fluid intelligence ability (for more detail about RAPM and its procedure, see Ref. 38). The details of RAPM are also mentioned in Chapter 7, 2D and 3D Educational Contents.

8.5.1.2 3D Visualization Material

In this study, stereoscopic 3D animations were used from Designmate, Inc., available at www.designnmate.com. The selected animations contained information about human anatomy and functions. Further, a 42-inch LG passive polarized 3D display with refresh rate 240 fps was used for visualization in this study.

8.5.1.3 Visual Oddball Task

The oddball paradigm is a commonly used task for cognitive and attention measurement in ERP studies.[38–40] In this study, two visual stimuli, a box and a sphere, shapes of size 5 cm, were designed as the standard and target stimuli, respectively (see Fig. 8.2). The presentation duration of each trial, either the standard (box) or target (sphere) trial, was 500 ms with the intertrial interval (ITI) between two consecutive trials being 500 ms. The participants were instructed to press "0" for a target stimulus and not to respond for a standard stimulus. Further, the reaction time and correct target detection of each participant were recorded. Two types of error were expected: false alarm (i.e., pressed key when standard stimulus was shown)

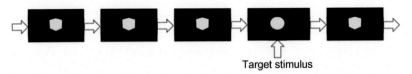

Target stimulus

Figure 8.2 Visual stimuli of oddball task[36] (box represents the standard stimulus and sphere represents the target stimulus).

and omission (forgot to press key when target stimulus appeared). Thirty percent of the trials were kept target and 70% were nontarget trials, i.e., there were 40 target trials and 135 total trials presented. Total time spent on the oddball task was 3.35 minutes.

8.5.2 Experiment Procedure

The EEG room used in the experimentation was partially sound-attenuated and each participant was briefed on the procedure. Then each participant attempted the RAPM test, which lasted 40 minutes. After the RAPM test, an EEG cap was set along with the PIB device (for ECG recording), which was followed by watching the stereoscopic 3D videos (2D group watched the videos in 2D mode and S3D group watched in 3D mode). The total duration of watching videos was 30 minutes. At the end of this session, participants performed the oddball task, which took approximately four minutes. For display, a 42-inch TV was used, placed at a distance of 1.5 m from the participant's sitting position. EEG signals were recorded during the learning session as well as during the oddball task using an EGI 128-channel net. The sampling rate was 250 points per second and the impedance of all the electrodes was kept below 50 kΩ (recommended by manufacturer) and referenced to the central electrode position Cz. ECG signals were recorded using the EGI Polygraphic Input Box (PIB). The FP1/FP2 electrodes were used to detect and extract the eye blinks from EEG recordings.

8.6 DATA DESCRIPTION

The E-Prime oddball task experiment is provided in the accompanying data files. The experiment design file can be opened and run with E-Prime software. The description of EEG and ERP data is provided in the following section.

8.6.1 EEG/ERP Description

EEG raw data, ERP clean data for single-trial analysis (nonaveraged data), and ERP averaged data, behavioral responses, and event files for one participant are provided with this chapter. The details of these files are provided in Table 8.1. To access these files, please go to the directory BookData\Chap08 in the data files accompanying this book. For the complete dataset of 68 participants, please contact the authors at brainexpbook@gmail.com.

Each participant's EEG recordings contain 135 trials including 40 target trials and 95 standard trials. The trials can be detected with the help of event files recorded in E-Prime software.[6] The event files contain the stimuli onset, offset, and response information synchronized with the EEG data. The preprocessing and ERP extraction procedures are reported in the papers listed in Section 8.7.

Table 8.1 Data files description

S. No.	Directory name	Description
01	EEG data	This directory contains the following EEG recordings: S1_eo.mat: Resting state EEG recording for eyes-closed condition. S1_eo.mat: Resting state EEG recording for eyes–open condition. S1_L1.mat: EEG recording during study session. In this recording, the participants watched animated learning contents while EEG data was recorded. S1_L2.mat and S1_L3.mat: In the EEG recording, the same animated contents (as shown in S1_L1.mat) were repeated to better memorize the learning material while EEG was recorded. The directory "EEG Data" contains another directory named "oddball data," in which two subfolders "Averaged ERP File" and "Non Averaged ERP File" are located. The former contains averaged ERP file "S1_avg.mat"; while the latter contains nonaveraged ERP file "S(1)_Oddball_st.mat" along with the event file "S(1)_oddball.evt." This event file contains events of stimulus onset (stm+) that can be used to segment nonaveraged EEG data for averaging or single-trial analysis. To this event information MATLAB code is provided to extract the events from the .evt file.

(Continued)

Table 8.1 Data files description (Continued)

S. No.	Directory name	Description
02	ECG data	This directory contains the ECG data recorded in parallel with the EEG data as described in S. No. 01. The following files are included in this directory: S1_EC.mat: Resting state ECG recording for eyes-closed condition. S1_EO.mat: ECG Recording during study session. In this recording the participants watched animated learning contents while ECG data was recorded. S1_L1.mat: ECG recording during study session. In this recording the participants watched animated learning contents while ECG data was recorded. S1_L2.mat and S1_L3.mat: In the ECG recording, the same animated contents (as shown in S1_L1.mat) were repeated to better memorize the learning material while ECG was recorded. S1_Oddball.mat: ECG recording during oddball task.
03	Behavioral data	This directory contains one participant's behavioral data. E-Prime creates .edat2 file against each time the experiment is run for each participant. The .edat2 file contains all the behavioral responses of the participant recorded during the experiment including stimulus onset, offset, reaction time, response key press, etc. One participant's .edat2 file is provided with the bookdata of this chapter.
04	Experiment	In the experiment directory, the designed oddball task in E-Prime ".es2 file" is provided along with stimuli. This file can be opened and run using E-Prime software.

8.6.2 Subjective Data Description

EGI Net Station software allows extracting different event files (.evt) from recorded EEG data. These events can contain information about eye blinks and eye movement artifacts that can be used during data preprocessing. In addition, events of stimulus onset, offset, feedback, and participant responses can be extracted from EEG data using Net Station, which can be used for EEG data segmentation, if the data is time locked. The event files can be opened in Microsoft Excel or read in MATLAB.

The E-Prime software creates a log file (.edat2) each time an E-Prime experiment runs. The log file records all the details of trials, participant information, session, session time, block, participants' correct and incorrect responses, reaction time, and onset/offset of stimulus. These log files can be opened in E-DataAid package of E-Prime software, and hardware dongle is not required. If E-Prime is not installed or the license is expired then the demo version (https://www.pstnet.com/demos/eprime/RequestDemo.aspx) can be downloaded; this will work for E-DataAid and the log file can be opened. Hence, the accuracy and reaction time of each participant can be computed from the .edat2 files using the predefined procedure in the E-Prime manual or can be exported to SPSS for statistical analysis.

8.7 RELEVANT PAPERS

This section provides a list of some of the papers that have utilized the data acquired from the experiment described in this chapter. The following papers should be cited when using the experiment design or the data provided with this chapter.

1. Amin HU, Malik AS, Badruddin N, Kamel N, Hussain M. Effects of stereoscopic 3D display technology on event-related potentials (ERPs). In: *7th International IEEE EMBS Conference on Neural Engineering*, Montpellier, France; 2015, pp. 1084–1087.

2. Amin HU, Malik AS, Mumtaz W, Badruddin N, Kamel N. Evaluation of passive polarized stereoscopic 3D display for visual & mental fatigues. In: *37th International IEEE EMBS Conference*, Melano, Italy; 2015, pp. 1084–1087.

ACKNOWLEDGMENTS

This chapter provides the details of the experiment design available in the papers mentioned in Section 8.7 and in the PhD thesis of Hafeez Ullah Amin, which is available at Universiti Teknologi PETRONAS.

REFERENCES

1. Malik AS, Raja Khairuddin RNH, Amin HU, et al. EEG based evaluation of stereoscopic 3D displays for viewer discomfort. *BioMed Eng OnLine.* 2015.
2. Li J, Barkowsky M, Le Callet P. Visual discomfort of stereoscopic 3D videos: influence of 3D motion. *Displays.* 2014;35(1):49–57.
3. Li HCO, Junho S, Keetaek K, Seunghyun L. Measurement of 3D Visual Fatigue Using Event-Related Potential (ERP): 3D Oddball Paradigm. *Paper presented at: 3DTV Conference: The True Vision—Capture, Transmission and Display of 3D Video*, May 28–30, 2008.

4. Kaneko K, Sakamoto K. Spontaneous blinks as a criterion of visual fatigue during prolonged work on visual display terminals. *Percept Mot Skills.* 2001;92(1):234–250.

5. Donghyun K, Sunghwan C, Sangil P, Kwanghoon S. Stereoscopic visual fatigue measurement based on fusional response curve and eye-blinks. *Paper presented at: Digital Signal Processing (DSP), 2011 17th International Conference on* July 6–8, 2011.

6. Amin HU, Malik AS, Badruddin N, Kamel N, Hussain M. Effects of stereoscopic 3D display technology on Event-related Potentials (ERPs). *Paper presented at: 7th International IEEE EMBS Conference on Neural Engineering; April 22–24th,* 2015; Montpellier, France.

7. Amin HU, Malik AS, Subhani AR, Badruddin N, Chooi W-T. Dynamics of scalp potential and autonomic nerve activity during intelligence test. Lee M, Hirose A, Hou Z-G, Kil R, editors. *Neural Information Processing,*Vol 8226. Berlin Heidelberg: Springer; 2013:9–16.

8. Tam WJ, Speranza F, Yano S, Shimono K, Ono H. Stereoscopic 3D-TV:Visual Comfort. *IEEE Trans Broadcast.* 2011;57(2):335–346.

9. McIntire JP, Havig PR, Geiselman EE. What is 3D good for? A review of human performance on stereoscopic 3D displays; 2012.

10. Kooi FL, Toet A. Visual comfort of binocular and 3D displays. *Displays.* 2004;25(2–3):99–108.

11. Javidi B, Okano F. *Three-dimensional television, video, and display technologies.* New York: Springer Science & Business Media; 2002.

12. Huang K,Yuan J-C, Tsai C-H, Hsueh W-J, Wang N-Y. How crosstalk affects stereopsis in stereoscopic displays. *Paper presented at: Electronic Imaging;* 2003.

13. Yano S, Ide S, Mitsuhashi T, Thwaites H. A study of visual fatigue and visual comfort for 3D HDTV/HDTV images. *Displays.* 2002;23(4):191–201.

14. Ukai K, Howarth PA. Visual fatigue caused by viewing stereoscopic motion images: Background, theories, and observations. *Displays.* 2008;29(2):106–116.

15. Li H-CO, Seo J, Kham K, Lee S. Measurement of 3D visual fatigue using event-related potential (ERP): 3D oddball paradigm. *Paper presented at: 2008 3DTV Conference: The True Vision-Capture, Transmission and Display of 3D Video;* 2008.

16. Ujike H, Watanabe H. Effects of stereoscopic presentation on visually induced motion sickness. *Paper presented at: IS&T/SPIE Electronic Imaging;* 2011.

17. Solimini AG. Are there side effects to watching 3D movies? A prospective crossover observational study on visually induced motion sickness. *PloS one.* 2013;8(2):e56160.

18. IJsselsteijn WA, de Ridder H, Vliegen J. Effects of stereoscopic filming parameters and display duration on the subjective assessment of eye strain. *Paper presented at: Electronic Imaging;* 2000.

19. Malik AS, Amin HU, Badruddin N, Kamel N, Ahmad RF, Mumtaz W. Evaluation of stereoscopic 3D based educational contents for long-term memorization. *Ann Neurol.* 2015;78(S19) S89-S89.

20. Malik AS, Amin HU, Kamel N, Chooi W-T, Hussain M. The effects of 3D technology on the brain during learning and memory recall processes. *Ann Neurol.* 2014;76 S24-S24.

21. Thomson WD. Eye problems and visual display terminals—the facts and the fallacies. *Ophthalmic Physiol Opt.* 1998;18(2):111–119.

22. Bergqvist U. Visual display terminal work—a perspective on long-term changes and discomforts. *Int J Ind Ergon.* 1995;16(3):201–209.

23. Ishida S, Yamashita Y, Matsuishi T, Ohshima M, Ohshima H, Maeda H. Photosensitive seizures provoked while viewing pocket monsters, a made-for-television animation program in Japan. *Paper presented at: EPILEPSIA;* 1999.

24. Abe M, Yoshizawa M, Sugita N, et al. Independent component analysis of finger photoplethysmography for evaluating effects of visually-induced motion sickness. *Paper presented at: International Conference on Virtual Reality;* 2007.

25. Shibata T, Kim J, Hoffman DM, Banks MS. The zone of comfort: predicting visual discomfort with stereo displays. *J Vision*. 2011;11(8):11.
26. Lambooij M, IJsselsteijn W, Heynderickx I. Visual discomfort of 3D TV: assessment methods and modeling. *Displays*. 2011;32(4):209–218.
27. Lambooij M, Fortuin M, Heynderickx I, IJsselsteijn W. Visual discomfort and visual fatigue of stereoscopic displays: a review. *J Imaging Sci Technol*. 2009;53(3) 30201-30201.
28. Kaseda Y, Jiang C, Kurokawa K, Mimori Y, Nakamura S. Objective evaluation of fatigue by event-related potentials. *J Neurol Sci*. 1998;158(1):96–100.
29. Polich J. Neuropsychology of P300. *Oxford handbook of event-related potential components*; 2012, pp. 159–188.
30. Mun S, Park M-C, Park S, Whang M. SSVEP and ERP measurement of cognitive fatigue caused by stereoscopic 3D. *Neurosci Lett*. 2012;525(2):89–94.
31. Murata A, Uetake A, Takasawa Y. Evaluation of mental fatigue using feature parameter extracted from event-related potential. *Int J Ind Ergon*. 2005;35(8):761–770.
32. Park S, Won M, Mun S, Lee E, Whang M. Does visual fatigue from 3D displays affect autonomic regulation and heart rhythm? *Int J Psychophysiol*. 2014;92(1):42–48.
33. Wronka E, Kaiser J, Coenen AML. Psychometric intelligence and P3 of the event-related potentials studied with a 3-stimulus auditory oddball task. *Neurosci Lett*. 2013;535(0):110–115.
34. Mun S, Kim E-S, Park M-C. Effect of mental fatigue caused by mobile 3D viewing on selective attention: an ERP study. *Int J Psychophysiol*. 2014;94(3):373–381.
35. Chen C-Y, Ke M-D, Wu P-J, Kuo C-D, Pong B-J, Lai Y-Y. The influence of polarized 3D display on autonomic nervous activities. *Displays*. 2014;35(4):196–201.
36. Amin HU, Malik AS, Mumtaz W, Badruddin N, Kamel N. Evaluation of passive polarized stereoscopic 3D display for visual & mental fatigues. *Paper presented at: Engineering in Medicine and Biology Society (EMBC), 2015 37th Annual International Conference of the IEEE*; August 25–29, 2015.
37. Portella C, Machado S, Arias-Carrión O, et al. Relationship between early and late stages of information processing: an event-related potential study. *Neurol Int*. 2012;4(3)
38. Amin HU, Malik AS, Kamel N, Chooi W-T, Hussain M. P300 correlates with learning & memory abilities and fluid intelligence. *J NeuroEng Rehabil*. 2015;12(1):87.
39. Huettel SA, McCarthy G. What is odd in the oddball task? Prefrontal cortex is activated by dynamic changes in response strategy. *Neuropsychologia*. 2004;42(3):379–386.
40. Maurage P, Philippot P, Verbanck P, et al. Is the P300 deficit in alcoholism associated with early visual impairments (P100, N170)? An oddball paradigm. *Clin Neurophysiol*. 2007;118(3):633–644.

CHAPTER 9

3D Video Games

Contents

9.1 INTRODUCTION

The popularity of gaming has increased in society. The traditional way of playing games uses two-dimensional (2D) technology. With the advancement in three-dimensional (3D) and virtual reality technologies, gamers are one of the first groups to embrace these technologies and are switching from 2D to 3D modes. However, the pros and cons of these technologies are not well studied. In addition to the technology involved, the effects of the content of the games are also not well researched; e.g., some may have positive effects while some may have negative effects on the human brain and ultimately human behavior.

The design of 2D games depends on sprites and drawings on a two-dimensional flat surface, while the 3D games depend on models and 3D shapes developed on a computer. Meanwhile, video games are evolving from traditional 2D to 3D and virtual reality technology; hence there is significant research potential to examine the brain's emotional activities during playing video games.[1] It is important because the game contents

Designing EEG Experiments for Studying the Brain.
DOI: http://dx.doi.org/10.1016/B978-0-12-811140-6.00009-6
© 2017 Elsevier Inc.
All rights reserved.
137

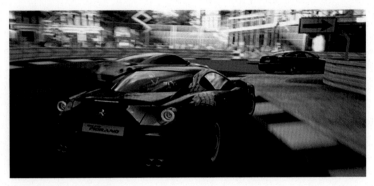

Figure 9.1 3D game interface.

have a connection with human behavior (see Fig. 9.1 for 3D game interface). Examples of video game content that may have adverse psychological effects include violence, sexual themes, substances, and profanity.[2]

The purpose of this experiment was to investigate the brain neuronal changes occurring due to playing video games and comparing the 2D and 3D modes during playing games. The neuronal changes of the brain were recorded by using electroencephalography (EEG) while playing the games. EEG is one of the imaging modalities that can be easily used to directly record the brain's electrical signals during any cognitive task. The recorded raw EEG signals can be analyzed to extract useful information for studying the brain using computational techniques.[3,4] Previous studies have investigated 3D technology for visual and mental fatigue and visual discomfort using EEG signals for 3D movies and 3D animated learning contents.[5,6]

The contents of the video games may be neutral, violence, aggression, or emotions. In one of the studies, video games were studied for the effect of violence and aggression. In one of the studies, the brain changes during playing games were recorded using the functional magnetic resonance imaging (fMRI) technique. The fMRI technique works on the principle of oxygen consumption in the blood. The amount of blood flow in the whole brain is determined via the magnetic responses of hemoglobin. However, the results of the study are questionable as the neural activity may not reflect aggressiveness due to violent action (which was reported), but rather fear of endangering the player's virtual life.[7]

9.2 IMPORTANCE OF STUDYING 3D VIOLENCE GAME

One of the core applications of stereoscopic 3D (S3D) technology is 3D video games. The S3D technology has enhanced the interest of the end users resulting in increased demand for video games in the entertainment market.[8] Video games require physical challenges on behalf of the players such as motor skills, coordination of eyes with hands, and mental alertness to respond in the limited amount of time.[9] Hence the brain is also required to be active and the working memory loaded with current information, planning of the next action in response to expected events, and decision making.

It has been shown that 3D video games have positive effects on the players' cognitive performance such as improvement in memory tasks.[10–12] All such positive effects are reported for normal and nonviolent 3D video games. Since violent 3D video games have also been developed, such as *Grand Theft Auto V* and *Killzone 3*, there is concern regarding the negative effects of violent 3D video games on players, especially children. It has been shown that violent 3D video games induce stress and anxiety,[13] as well as increase aggressive thoughts,[14,15] motivation toward violence,[16,17] and game addiction.[18]

Because playing 3D video games is common in children and young adults, the impact of violent 3D video games is critical to explore and determine the causes of or find ways to control the level of violence in these video games. The previous research that reported the negative effects of 3D video games, such as stress and anxiety, aggressive thoughts, and/or motivation toward violence, are based on behavior investigations. However, it is not clear how brain neuronal networks are altered by the contents of 3D violent video games in order to cause negative changes in the behavior of the players. Therefore the use of EEG will unfold the neuronal activities affected due to playing violent 3D video games and the changes in the specific EEG pattern that may cause the negative behaviors of the players. It may be possible to determine the specific EEG pattern changes due to playing 3D violent video games and then adopt treatment such as neurofeedback therapy to recover the EEG pattern to normal conditions and avoid the development of negative behaviors in the players.

9.3 PROBLEM STATEMENT

Various video gaming content that may have adverse psychological effects includes violence, sexual themes, substances, and profanity. The development of 3D-based video games and the popularity of 3D technology is rapidly growing. There is a risk for the human brain to be affected due to such circumstances where the contents of the video games include

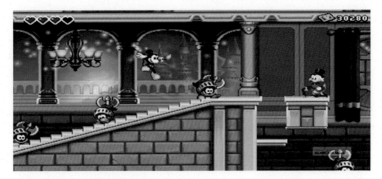

Figure 9.2 Interface of 2D game.

violence. Hence the following main research objectives were covered in this experiment:

1. To investigate the effects of 2D- and 3D-based video game technologies on the human brain.
2. To examine the brain for the effects of video games with violent content on EEG signals.

9.4 DESCRIPTION OF 2D- AND 3D-BASED VIDEO GAMES

Today advanced video game contents are available in different varieties and with different technologies in the market. Apart from the differences in the contents, there are major differences regarding the display modes, i.e., 2D or 3D video games. The 2D games are also referred as platform games in which the visual objects and characters are cartoonish and unrealistic (see Fig. 9.2 for 2D game interface).[19] The character can be viewed only from one perspective, i.e., from the side view, top view, or player's eye view. Besides that, 2D computer graphics are digital images where a simple picture or some matte painting image for background is used.[20]

The 3D-based video games provide a sense of realism with depth perception, attracting more attention and emotions. The players may be more involved in the games, with high attention and greater use of cognitive resources of the brain compared to the traditional 2D games. In 3D games, the player is allowed to move the camera in three dimensions. The features of 3D vision, including lighting, shadows, and depth, can be rendered with computer software such as 3DS Max.[20]

9.5 SOFTWARE AND HARDWARE TOOLS

A description of the equipment and software tools used in this experiment is provided in Table 9.1.

Table 9.1 Equipment and software description

S. No.	Item	Description
01	EEG 20-channel Enobio system	This EEG system was developed by StarLab, Barcelona, Spain. This is a wearable and wireless 20-channel EEG system ideal for research application and covers the 10–20 system. The acquisition software has a user-friendly interface for easy configuration, recording, and visualization. For more details, see http://www.neuroelectrics.com/
02	PlayStation 3 player and console	The PlayStation 3 system is a home video game console produced by Sony. The PlayStation 3 controller was also used for the video game. This system was employed for the experiment in this study https://www.playstation.com/en-us/explore/ps3/
03	3D active television	40-in. Sony 3D active TV was used for displaying the video game http://www.sony.com/
04	Sony 3D active shutter glasses	These glasses were used to achieve immersive realism while playing the video games with PlayStation 3 and the 3D active TV
05	*Killzone 3* CD game	This is a 3D video game for the PlayStation 3 launched by Sony in 2011. The game can be played using a stereoscopic 3D display and the PlayStation Move motion-sensing controller to achieve more immersive realism. https://www.playstation.com/en-us/games/killzone-3-ps3/

(Continued)

Table 9.1 Equipment and software description (Continued)

S. No.	Item	Description
06	EEGLAB MATLAB toolbox	Delorme & Makeig developed EEGLAB, an open source free toolbox-based MATLAB platform in 2004 for analysis of EEG and MEG data analysis. EEGLAB allows the user to load EEG/MEG raw data, as well as process, visualize, and perform artifact removal using ICA and/or manual rejection. This toolbox was used for data cleaning and analysis http://sccn.ucsd.edu/eeglab/

9.6 EXPERIMENTAL DESIGN AND PROTOCOL

9.6.1 Target Population

In this study, the students on the university campus were the target population. These were the possible respondents that may fulfill the required criteria for participant recruitment. All the students on the university campus were the entire set of units for which the findings of the research had been generalized. Three levels of students were studying on the campus at the time of data collection, i.e., foundation level, undergraduate level, and postgraduate level. Equal opportunity was given to all students who met the inclusion criteria to become a participant.

9.6.2 Inclusion Criteria

The inclusion criteria are essential for all the participants to meet prior to joining the experiment.

The requirements were:
- Participant should be between 18 and 25 years in age
- Participant should be right-handed
- Participant should be a beginner (mastery level of playing games)
- Participant must be physically and mentally healthy (normal or corrected vision, no major medical issues or head injuries)

9.6.3 Exclusion Criteria

The exclusion criteria are the requirements used for exclusion of partici-pants from this study. The participants were excluded in this experiment when they:

- Failed to meet the criteria of written consent
- Failed to meet the criteria mentioned in the inclusion list

9.6.4 Sample Size Computation

The sample size of computation for this study was not predefined because this was a pilot study. Further research on this topic may be needed to properly compute the sample size using the mean differences among the three groups of this study, which were reported in the final year project (FYP) report available at UTP Institutional Repository (http://eprints. utp.edu.my/).

9.6.5 Experimental Video Game Contents

There are many types of content in video games that may have adverse psychological effects, namely, violence, sexual themes, substances, and profanity. In this project, violent content was selected by using the game *Killzone 3*. Violence is defined as "acts in which the aggressor causes or attempts to cause physical injury or death to another character."[2] Each violent scene was counted once with the following circumstances:

- continuous attack with violent acts
- when a character hit the opponent multiple times in an attack with violent magic or spinning attack, etc.
- condition of many characters such as group battle

The level of violence in video games is measured by the amount of blood existing in the game. In video games, the blood that reflects the violence is defined as "a red fluid originating from an injured human or any color fluid originating from an injured creature." The level of blood is coded as "animated blood," realistic blood," or "blood and gore."[21]

In this project, a violent video game was used. However, there are video games that have contents such as sexual themes, substances, and pro-fanity. In games with sexual themes, the sexuality traits include the size and shape of the body character, the attire, and the parts of exposure. Drugs, alcohol, tobacco, and gambling comprise the addictive substances and behavior category. Lastly, one of the video contents is the practice of profanity in song lyrics, either spoken or written. It is considered that profanity is the "use of abusive and vulgar language and obscene gestures." [21]

9.6.6 Experiment Design and Procedure

The experiment consisted of a total of three sessions. In the first session, the participants were asked to fill out a questionnaire (see Appendix 9A) with questions about the participant's experience in playing video games and health-related questions such as medical history and present status of health. Once it was confirmed by the experimenter that the participant did not have any health issues that may go against the study's objectives or the inclusion criteria then the participant was asked to read the research information (see Appendix 14) and sign the informed consent (see Appendix 2C). After signing the consent form, they were asked to move on to the second session.

In the second session, the participant was asked to practice the violent video games to get familiar with the procedure and rules of play before the actual experimentation. The participants played the video games both in 2D modes and 3D modes alternately. Each participant did 30 minutes practice in this session. When the practice session was completed, the participants were asked to appear in the third session the next day.

In the third session, an electrode cap was placed on the participant's head. The duration of cap fitting was about 15–20 minutes. During EEG recording, they were asked to perform four tasks. In the first task, they watched a cross "X" with white background paper for 5 minutes. The first 5 minutes of EEG recording is used as baseline signal and for analysis of the artifacts in EEG. In the second task, the participants were given 20 minutes to practice the game in 2D. During this practice, the participants were required to know how to play the game. In the third task, they started playing the games in 2D for 30 minutes. The EEG signals were recorded during the last 5 minutes of playing. Finally, for the fourth task, they played the games in 3D for 30 minutes and their EEG signals were recorded during the last 5 minutes of game playing. All tasks were completed in approximately 100 minutes. There was a 5-minute break at regular intervals to rest. This experiment was completed in 2 days.

9.7 EXPERIMENTAL DATA ACCOMPANYING THIS CHAPTER

EEG raw and clean data for one subject are provided with this book. The details of these files are provided in Table 9.2. To access these files, please

Table 9.2 EEG data description

S. No.	File name	Description
01	EO.edf	Five minutes EEG recording for baseline eyes-open condition before watching the video games
02	3D.edf	Five minutes EEG recording during playing the video games using 3D active shutter glasses
03	2D.edf	Five minutes EEG recording during playing the video games in 2D mode

go to the directory BookData\Chapter9\clean for preprocessed data and BookData\Chap9\raw for raw data in the data files accompanying this book. For the complete dataset of 23 subjects, please contact the authors at brainexpbook@gmail.com.

9.8 RELEVANT PAPERS

This section provides a list of some of the papers that have utilized the data acquired from the experiment described in this chapter. The following papers should be cited when using the experiment design or the data provided with this chapter.

1. Malik AS, Alif A, Osman DA, Hamizah RN. Disparity in brain dynamics for video games played on small and large displays. *IEEE Symposium on Humanities, Science & Engineering Research (SHUSER)*. Kuala Lumpur, Malaysia; June 24–27, 2012: 1067–1071.

2. Malik AS, Osman DA, Alif A, Hamizah RN. Investigating brain activation with respect to playing video games on large screens. *International Conference on Intelligent and Advanced Systems (ICIAS), Conference Proceedings 1, art. no. 6306165*; Kuala Lumpur, Malaysia: June 12–14, 2012, 86–90.

ACKNOWLEDGMENTS

This chapter provides the details of the experiment design available in the papers mentioned in Section 9.8 and in the BS FYP report of Shazlin Afiza Binti Sopian, which is available at Universiti Teknologi PETRONAS.

REFERENCES

1. Sheikholeslami C, Yuan H, He EJ, Bai X, Yang L, He B. A high resolution EEG study of dynamic brain activity during video game play. *Paper presented at: Engineering in Medicine and Biology Society, 2007. EMBS 2007. 29th Annual International Conference of the IEEE 2007.*

2. Haninger K, Thompson KM. Content and ratings of teen-rated video games. *JAMA*. 2004;291(7):856–865.
3. Amin HU, Malik AS, Kamel N, Hussain M. A novel approach based on data redundancy for feature extraction of EEG signals. *Brain Topogr*. 2016;29(2):207–217.
4. Amin HU, Malik AS, Ahmad RF, et al. Feature extraction and classification for EEG signals using wavelet transform and machine learning techniques. *Australas Phys Eng Sci Med*. 2015;38(1):139–149.
5. Amin HU, Malik AS, Mumtaz W, Badruddin N, Kamel N. Evaluation of passive polarized stereoscopic 3D display for visual & mental fatigues. *Paper presented at: Engineering in Medicine and Biology Society (EMBC), 2015. 37th Annual International Conference of the IEEE*; August 25–29, 2015.
6. Malik AS, Khairuddin RNHR, Amin HU, et al. EEG based evaluation of stereoscopic 3D displays for viewer discomfort. *BioMed Eng OnLine*. 2015;14(1):21.
7. Weber R, Ritterfeld U, Mathiak K. Does playing violent video games induce aggression? Empirical evidence of a functional magnetic resonance imaging study. *Media Psychol*. 2006;8(1):39–60.
8. Zhu F, Zhang X. The influence of online consumer reviews on the demand for experience goods: The case of video games. *ICIS 2006 Proceedings*. 2006:25.
9. Wolf MJ, Perron B. *The Video Game Theory Reader*. : Psychology Press; 2003.
10. Spence I, Feng J. Video games and spatial cognition. *Rev Gen Psychol*. 2010;14(2):92.
11. Cockburn A, McKenzie B. Evaluating the effectiveness of spatial memory in 2D and 3D physical and virtual environments. *Paper presented at: Proceedings of the SIGCHI Conference on Human factors in Computing Systems 2002*.
12. Gee JP. *What Video Games Have to Teach Us About Learning and Literacy*. Macmillan; 2014.
13. Bouchard S, Bernier F, Boivin É, et al. Modes of immersion and stress induced by commercial (off-the-shelf) 3D games. *J Def Model Simul*. 2012;11(4):339–352.
14. Carnagey NL, Anderson CA, Bushman BJ. The effect of video game violence on physiological desensitization to real-life violence. *J Exp Soc Psychol*. 2007;43(3):489–496.
15. Adachi PJC, Willoughby T. The effect of violent video games on aggression: is it more than just the violence? *Aggress Violent Behav*. 2011;16(1):55–62.
16. Ferguson CJ, Rueda SM, Cruz AM, Ferguson DE, Fritz S, Smith SM. Violent video games and aggression causal relationship or byproduct of family violence and intrinsic violence motivation? *Crim Justice Behav*. 2008;35(3):311–332.
17. Ravaja N, Turpeinen M, Saari T, Puttonen S, Keltikangas-Järvinen L. The psychophysiology of James Bond: phasic emotional responses to violent video game events. *Emotion*. 2008;8(1):114.
18. Yee N. Motivations for play in online games. *CyberPsychol Behav*. 2006;9(6):772–775.
19. Chang A. Ezine Articles. 2013; <http://ezinearticles.com>. Accessed February 16, 2013.
20. Myer C. SelfGrowth.com. 2013; <http://www.selfgrowth.com>. Accessed February 16, 2013.
21. Robinson T, Callister M, Clark B, Phillips J. Violence, sexuality, and gender stereotyping: a content analysis of official video game web sites. *Web J Mass Commun Res*. 2008;13:1–17.

CHAPTER 10

Visually Induced Motion Sickness

Contents

10.1 INTRODUCTION

Stereoscopy is the illusion of creating depth in two-dimensional (2D) images. The technique of stereoscopy is based on binocular vision, i.e., viewing two images at the same time, which gives a perception of depth. Human perception of three dimensions is based on a number of cues such as binocular parallax, motion parallax, accommodation, and convergence.

The advancements in display technology have taken this to a new dimension. Display technology is now moving from 2D viewing to 3D viewing. Adding another dimension to display devices increases the entertainment value to viewers, since images seem more realistic and life-like and appear to "pop out" from the TV screen. The entertainment and film industries continue to explore new and exciting ways of filmmaking and producing animations in 3D. The audiences too are showing more interest in films and animations that incorporate the latest viewing experiences.

Designing EEG Experiments for Studying the Brain.
DOI: http://dx.doi.org/10.1016/B978-0-12-811140-6.00010-2
© 2017 Elsevier Inc.
All rights reserved.
147

Hence they are more likely to enjoy films that offer an immersive feeling where the audience feels like they are part of the scenes.

The popularity of 3D technology is found in entire world but this technology is not limited to entertainment only; instead it is moving into different fields, whether that is medical science, sports, or even lectures of primary students. Now content can be found in 3D stereoscopy. The growth of 3D technology assures us that in future, viewing devices will have additional feature of 3D in them. It can be assumed that large screen TVs, computer screens, smart phones, and tablet PCs all will be converted to 3D soon. Every new cinema shows 3D movies and almost every month there is a new 3D movie in the market that people are eager to watch.

By the end of 2009, Sony announced that it will be bringing 3D viewing into home viewing environment and experts claimed that "we will watch all our media in 3D within a decade." Sony's chairman Howard Stringer said that 3D will be the next $10 billion business.[1] Other companies have also joined the 3D bandwagon, with the president of Samsung Electronics' visual display division, Mr. Yoon Boo-Keun, announcing "Samsung aims to sell 2 million 3D LED TVs in 2010".[2] At present, there are a number of 3D TV choices available in the market, and most of them use either active or passive glasses.

10.1.1 Types of Stereoscopy

Different methods are used to produce stereoscopic effect. They can be classified into aided viewing or free viewing. Aided viewing is further divided into active and passive. Passive includes anaglyph and polarized glasses while active includes liquid crystal display (LCD) shutter glasses. Auto stereoscopic display, which does not require any filtering lenses, is known for free viewing.

- Anaglyph: These are also called color-multiplexed displays. In anaglyphs, the two right and left images are filtered with colors like red and green, red and cyan, and green and magenta. The viewers have to wear the same filter lenses, which produce the effect of 3D depth in the images.
- Polarized glasses: In polarized glasses, each lens is perpendicularly polarized. Therefore, the eyes see the image based on horizontal and vertical polarized light. The effect of 3D in polarized glasses is better than in anaglyphs.
- LCD shutter glasses: Shutter glasses are electronically powered and one lens of the glass is active at a time. They are synchronized with the

refresh rate of the screen. The display device displays only one image and this gets synced with the lens; therefore, the eyes are intended to see only particular frames that create the depth effect.

- Auto stereoscopic displays: Auto stereo displays are a more advanced form of stereoscopy. In auto stereo, multiple views of an object are created from multiple cameras. Frames are presented on the screen with left and right views parallel to each other. The views are set in a way that left and right eyes can see their respective frames only. Parallax barrier and lenticular lens are two different modes of producing auto stereoscopic images.

From the aspects of entertainment and enjoyment, viewers find stereoscopic displays to be the best viewing device to give themselves a feeling of immersion. Viewers enjoy being a part of the movies they are watching as the things fly by them and motion looks more realistic. Even 3D stereoscopy has provided much entertainment to viewers but some viewers suffer from side effects of this technology. Viewers have reported that after watching 3D stereoscopic films they feel strain in their eyes and it gives them a headache. Based on the interviews of viewers, an article reports that 3D might be the cause of altered vision, confusion, and dizziness.[3] It is also reported from an ophthalmologist that people with minor imbalance in their eyes can have a headache while watching 3D movies.[4] These symptoms are derived from motion sickness, and the type of motion sickness that is caused by viewing is known as visually induced motion sickness (VIMS).

10.2 IMPORTANCE OF STUDYING VIMS FOR 3D DISPLAYS

The research studies investigating viewers' complaints and symptoms of dissatisfaction with respect to stereoscopy vision reported the common issues faced by the viewers during watching stereoscopic 3D contents (either movies or games), such as dizziness, disorientation, headache, visual and mental fatigue, visual discomfort, eye strain, and so on.[5,6] In addition, it is also known that not all viewers report the same symptoms. A viewer who is suffering from these symptoms will have VIMS, which is a condition where viewers are being physically still during or after exposure to 3D content but they feel symptoms of VIMS.[7]

A well-known standard tool for assessment of VIMS is the simulator sickness questionnaire (SSQ), which is a structure questionnaire reported in previous research for subjective judgment of VIMS.[7,8] Since the SSQ allows subjective assessment of VIMS, there are limitations of the subjective assessment reported in previous research such as systematic and cognitive biasness[9] and psychological factors,[10] often negatively correlated with the variable of interest[11,12] and difficult to interpret because they are often expressed in ordinal scales.[13] Therefore, an EEG method is adopted in the experiment described in this chapter along with the SSQ tool to measure the EEG waves, which directly reflect the electrical activity of the brain.

The assessment of VIMS is important because the use of S3D technology is spread out in many disciplines other than entertainment, such as education. In the education sector, the learning of science concepts is supported by the use of S3D animation for understanding and easy memorization.[14,15] Hence, such a research study will explore the side effects of S3D technology such as VIMS and the possible factors that cause such symptoms.

10.3 PROBLEM STATEMENT AND OBJECTIVES

3D stereoscopic technology is growing day-by-day with advancements in hardware as well as in content. Viewers look at 3D as the future of display devices. If problems of VIMS persist in 3D stereoscopy, viewers might be struck by VIMS or certain symptoms of VIMS. This will ruin the entertainment of the viewers, and they will have to pay for unexpected costs. Therefore it is necessary to evaluate the symptoms of VIMS that are produced by 3D stereoscopy. These symptoms should be compared to a normal 2D display device. The symptoms should be recorded, analyzed, and compared between the two devices. Based on the comparative analysis, symptoms of VIMS in 3D could be adjudged.

For the evaluation of VIMS, it is important to know that how VIMS can be easily induced and evaluated. Evaluation of VIMS requires different methods that can be subjective (questionnaire or interviews) and objective (physiological data). A combination of different data provides a suitable outcome. In this study, the SSQ in combination with electrocardiography (ECG) and electroencephalography (EEG) signals were recorded for the comparative analysis of 3D display with 2D display. EEG signals directly measure the neuronal changes occurring due to VIMS or cognitive fatigue and can be quantitatively analyzed using computational techniques to determine useful information for assessment of brain states.[16,17] Similarly, ECG signals that refer to the dynamics of heartbeats are useful to study the heart rate variability (HRV) during any mental state such as visual discomfort.[18]

The experiment was designed with the following objectives:

- To find the brain regions that are activated when VIMS is present.
- To evaluate and compare the brain wave changes and level of motion sickness in individuals induced by 2D and 3D movies.
- To propose an objective indicator/measurement of VIMS using EEG signals.

10.4 VISUALLY INDUCED MOTION SICKNESS

Previously several studies reported different symptoms due to watching stereoscopy videos/games such as visual fatigue, visual discomfort, eye strain, blurred vision, headache, dizziness, confusion, and disorientation.[19–22] There are differences among people's feedback regarding the symptoms; in other words, not all people reported the same symptoms. Therefore, an individual experiencing such symptoms is considered as suffering from VIMS. This situation is categorized as a type of Cinerama sickness in which visual signals are present but signals from the vestibular system are absent.[23]

There are four main mechanisms responsible for depth in the human visual system, i.e., binocular parallax, motion parallax, accommodation, and convergence.[24] The 3D stereoscopic technology uses disparity between images to produce depth, which is one of these mechanisms. The disparity can be categorized as positive (uncrossed) disparity, in which objects are at the back of screen and negative (crossed) disparity where the objects are in front of the screen. It has been reported that vergence is more active in 3D movies than in 2D.[25] The disparity present in the visual scene causes the vergence and henceforth the eye will go through accommodation. In the accommodation process, the lens adjusts itself to focus the light beams on the fovea; consequently if the eyes produce vergence, accommodation will spontaneously take place. It has been reported that the main reason for visual fatigue is a conflict in vergence and accommodation response. Vergence and accommodation have their own limits that cause the problems in vision.

In a real-world scene, the accommodation and vergence point coincides no matter where the viewer looks. The accommodation and vergence responses are coupled and accommodative changes evoke vergences and vice versa. The benefit of coupling is the increased speed of accommodation and vergence. However, this has not happened in the case of 3D stereoscopy. In 3D displays, the correlation between focal and vergence distance is disrupted, i.e., the focal distance is fixed at the display while the vergence distance changes depending on the simulated visual scene the observer fixates.

Such problems with 3D technology cause discomfort in viewing. Users of 3D technology who are intolerant to the previously mentioned discomforts may experience VIMS. In previous studies, visual stress and symptoms of VIMS are reported during and after watching a 3D movie.[26] It is also reported that children must be cautioned when exposed to 3D TV, because they may not be able to realize any physical problem even if it exists.[27] Furthermore, 5% of viewers in 3D cinemas experience symptoms of nausea or disorientation.[28]

10.4.1 Methods of Inducing Motion Sickness

Motion sickness is defined as a conflict between the visual system and vestibular system—the sensory system in humans used to maintain a sense of balance and spatial orientation.[29] Therefore, motion sickness may be induced by creating such a conflict in any of the two senses. Three possibilities can occur when there are conflicts in visual and vestibular cues. The first possibility is that both visual and vestibular cues are present but are giving conflicting information to the brain. In the other two possibilities, either visual or vestibular cues are absent. If visual signals are present and vestibular signals are absent, then this kind of motion sickness is mostly caused by viewing motion in a stationary environment. The symptoms are not very severe, but they can cause motion sickness. If the vestibular signal is present and visual signal is absent, this scenario is almost the opposite of the first case with stationary visual gaze and moving environment. For example, reading during a moving journey can cause this type of motion sickness.

10.5 SOFTWARE AND HARDWARE

The following software and hardware were used in the collection and organization of this dataset:

1. Electrical Geodesics, Inc. (128-channel EEG equipment with Net Station software)
2. LG stereoscopic TV with 3D glasses
3. TOBII Eye Tracker and software
4. MATLAB 2010 (for simulation)
5. PASS for sample size calculation
6. SPSS for statistical analysis

10.6 EXPERIMENTAL DESIGN AND PROTOCOL

10.6.1 Study Population

Students from Universiti Teknologi PETRONAS were recruited for selection in the experiment. The study was based on the following reference:
- Students who were willing to participate and fill out their consent to take part in the experiment.
- Students who fulfilled selection criteria.

The experiment was conducted in the Centre of Intelligent Signal and Imaging Research (CISIR), Universiti Teknologi PETRONAS, during the months of November and December 2012.

10.6.2 Sample Size Computation

Sample size formula:

$$n = f(\alpha, P)\left(\frac{p_1(1 - p_1) \times p_2(1 - p_2)}{(p_1 - p_2)^2}\right)$$

a = significance level, 0.05
P = power of the study, 80%
p_1 = probability of motion sickness in 2D case, 18.5% fixed base simulators[30]
p_2 = probability of motion sickness in 3D case, 59.1%[31]
n = 21 participants for one group
Participants were allocated to 2D and 3D by stratified sampling method. The number of female participants was proportionally less than male participants. Therefore, to remove a gender bias from the study, stratified sampling was implemented. Through stratified sampling, the proportion of males and females in both the groups were equal; this was done using SPSS software.

10.6.3 Selection Criteria

10.6.3.1 Inclusion Criteria

The following were the inclusion criteria for the participants:
- Subject from 18 to 40 years of age having normal refraction, i.e., emmetropia (+1.00 D and −0.25 D) or corrected to normal vision.[32] An ophthalmologist checked the eyesight of each participant before starting the experiment. The checkup included visual

acuity, refraction, and fundus examination. See Appendix 10A for the examination chart.

- Subjects whose susceptibility score is less than 30 as determined by the Motion Sickness Susceptibility Questionnaire (MSSQ).[33] See Appendix 10B for MSSQ.

10.6.3.2 Exclusion Criteria

The following are the exclusion criteria for the participants:

- Individuals who have seen 3D movies within 3 months of the experiment.
- Subjects with refractive error, i.e., myopia, hyperopia, and presbyopia.
- Subjects with eye diseases such as glaucoma, retinal or corneal disorder.
- Subjects with history of eye surgery such as cataract surgery, cornea, or retinal surgery.
- Subjects with history of eye injury or trauma.
- Subjects with any head injury or neurological disease like epilepsy, seizures, and migraine.
- Subjects with systemic problems such as hypertension, diabetes mellitus, asthma, and heart disease.
- Subjects with any ear problems or surgery.

10.6.4 Experiment Design

From the literature, it is clear that 3D produces symptoms of VIMS that can vary from one person to another. The symptoms that are mostly induced are visual and related to the occulomotor system, such as visual fatigue, eye strain, headache, etc. VIMS is not limited to these symptoms; other symptoms like disorientation and nausea can be found. For this purpose we designed an experiment that would induce motion sickness by watching a movie. The movie selected for the experiment was specially created to induce VIMS in participants.[34] The points considered during the experiment design are as follows:

- A large screen 3D TV to display the stimulus. Viewing on a large screen prompts viewers to have a feeling of involvement in the scene, and they feel more symptoms of VIMS.[35]
- Stimulus used was animated with specialized movements to induce VIMS. This reduces the time of the experiment, as a normal movie viewing would take more time to induce symptoms of VIMS and the symptoms induced can be rated on a reasonable scale.
- EEG and ECG were recorded as the objective parameters while SSQ was taken at the end to compare the subjective rating.

- EEG was selected as the major recording parameter because it records brains neuronal activity with high temporal resolution.
- Within EEG a dense array EEG device with 128 channels was selected so that brain activity with higher spatial resolution can be achieved.
- Participants were asked to give written consent before participating in the study. See Appendix 2C for the consent form.
- Maximum duration for the experiment was two hours and participants were compensated for the time spent.

The experiment flow chart is presented in Fig. 10.1.

10.6.4.1 Visual Stimulus

A passive polarized 42-inch 3D LCD TV was used for stimulus presentation. The visual stimulus was shown using TOBII software. The visual stimulus was a video that moves along a road, showing a view of movement (Fig. 10.2). Specialized movements along pitch and roll axes were created in the animated video (the visual stimulus). The animated video was created in such a way that the camera was rotated alternately on the two axes with 30 degrees of amplitude and 0.167 Hz of temporal frequency. Both the 2D and 3D versions of the animated video were created using 3D computer graphics software (Omega Space, Solidray Inc.).

A previous study had shown that with camera rotations along the pitch and roll axes, VIMS can be easily induced.[36] The duration of the animated

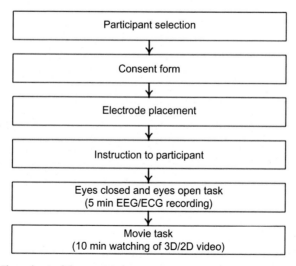

Figure 10.1 Flow chart of the experiment.

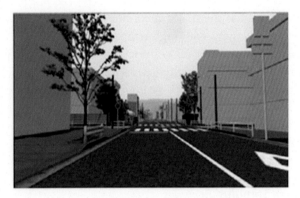

Figure 10.2 A view of the stimulus as seen by the participants.

video was two minutes. The animated video consisted of rotation along the pitch axis in the first minute, and in the second minute, the rotation was along the roll axis. In the experiment, the animated video was repeated five times, making the total duration 10 minutes.

10.7 EXPERIMENT DATA ACCOMPANYING THIS BOOK

In this experiment, Electrical Geodesic Inc. (EGI) HydroCel Geodesic Sensor Net with 128-channel EEG device was employed for EEG recording. The net was prepared with saline electrolyte to minimize impedance and improve quality of signals. In the recording, 250 samples per second was used as the sampling rate. The EEG raw data was recorded and stored on the hard disk drive as backup for further analysis. A notch filter was used to remove line noise of 50 Hz. Average referencing was used during the recoding.

EEG, ECG, and SSQ data for one subject are provided with this book in a separate directory. To access these files, please go to the directory BookData\Chap10\ in the data files accompanying this book. The details of these files are provided in Table 10.1. For the complete dataset of 42 subjects, please contact the authors at brainexpbook@gmail.com.

10.8 RELEVANT PAPERS

This section provides a list of some of the papers that have utilized the data acquired from the experiment described in this chapter. The

Table 10.1 EEG and ECG data description

S. No.	Directory name	Description
01	Eyesclosed	This directory contains eyes-closed EEG or ECG 5 minutes resting state recording of one participant. The name is "EC" and it is in .mat file format. The EEG and ECG data are provided in separate directories.
02	Eyesopen	This directory contains eyes-open EEG or ECG 5 minutes resting state recording of one participant. The name is "EO" and it is in .mat file format. The EEG and ECG data are provided in separate directories.
03	VIMS	This directory contains 10 minutes EEG or ECG recording during watching the movie with VIMS stimuli. The EEG and ECG data are provided in separate directories.
04	SSQ	This directory contains the SSQ responses of one subject recording via questionnaire and saved as an Excel spreadsheet. Computing SSQ grades: There are total items 1–16 (scale of 0–3) in the SSQ. Nausea (items 1, 6, 7, 8, 9, 15, 16), Oculomotor (items 1 to 5, 9, and 11), and Disorientation (items 5, 8, and 10–14). Scale multiplication factor: Nausea: A = score × 9.54; Oculomotor: B = score × 7.58; Disorientation: C = score × 13.92; Total SSQ score = $(A + B + C)$ × 3.74

following papers should be cited when using the experiment design or the data provided with this chapter.

1. Naqvi SAA, Badruddin N, Jatoi MA, Malik AS, Hazabbah W, Abdullah B. EEG based time and frequency dynamics analysis of visually induced motion sickness (VIMS). *Australas Phys Eng Sci Med*. 2015;38: 721–729.
2. Naqvi SAA, Badruddin N, Malik AS, Hazabbah W, Abdullah B. Does 3D produce more symptoms of visually induced motion sickness? In: *Engineering in Medicine and Biology Society (EMBC), 2013 35th Annual International Conference of the IEEE*, 2013;pp. 6405–6408.

ACKNOWLEDGMENTS

This chapter provides the details of the experiment design available in the papers mentioned in Section 10.8 and in the MSc thesis of Syed Ali Arslan Naqvi, which is available at Universiti Teknologi PETRONAS.

REFERENCES

1. Yasu M, Shiraki M. Sony's Stringer Sees 3D as Next $10 Billion Business. <http://www.bloomberg.com/apps/news?pid=newsarchive&sid=adp8a7FrDg.E>; 2009 Accessed March 9, 2012; 2011.
2. Yoo-chul K. Samsung Aims to Sell 2 Mil. 3D TVs in 2010. <http://www.koreatimes.co.kr/www/news/tech/2011/03/129_61416.html>; 2010 Accessed March 9, 2012; 2012.
3. Hurst D. How watching 3D films can be bad for your brain. <http://www.dailymail.co.uk/health/article-1271618/How-watching-3D-films-bad-brain.html>; 2010 Accessed December 12, 2011; 2011.
4. Steenhuysen J. 3D movies a headache for some. <http://www.abc.net.au/science/articles/2010/01/11/2789551.htm>; 2010 Accessed December 23, 2011; 2011.
5. Kooi FL, Toet A. Visual comfort of binocular and 3D displays. *Displays*. 2004; 25(2–3):99–108.
6. Javidi B, Okano F. *Three-Dimensional Television, Video, and Display Technologies*. New York: Springer Science & Business Media; 2002.
7. Wibirama S, Hamamoto K. Investigation of visually induced motion sickness in dynamic 3D contents based on subjective judgment, heart rate variability, and depth gaze behavior. *Paper presented at: 2014 36th Annual International Conference of the IEEE Engineering in Medicine and Biology Society*; August 26–30, 2014.
8. Kennedy RS, Lane NE, Berbaum KS, Lilienthal MG. Simulator sickness questionnaire: an enhanced method for quantifying simulator sickness. *Int J Aviat Psychol*. 1993;3(3):203–220.
9. Podsakoff PM, MacKenzie SB, Lee J-Y, Podsakoff NP. Common method biases in behavioral research: a critical review of the literature and recommended remedies. *J Appl Psychol*. 2003;88(5):879.
10. Bertrand M, Mullainathan S. Do people mean what they say? Implications for subjective survey data. *Am Econ Rev*. 2001;91(2):67–72.
11. Olken BA. Corruption perceptions vs. corruption reality. *J Public Econ*. 2009;93(7):950–964.
12. Razafindrakoto M, Roubaud F. Are international databases on corruption reliable? A comparison of expert opinion surveys and household surveys in Sub-Saharan Africa. *World Dev*. 2010;38(8):1057–1069.
13. Rose-Ackerman S, Palifka BJ. *Corruption and Government: Causes, Consequences, and Reform*. Cambridge: Cambridge University Press; 2016.
14. Malik AS, Amin HU, Badruddin N, Kamel N, Ahmad RF, Mumtaz W. Evaluation of stereoscopic 3D based educational contents for long-term memorization. *Ann Neurol*. 2015;78(S19):S89–S89.
15. Malik AS, Amin HU, Kamel N, Chooi W-T, Hussain M. The effects of 3D technology on the brain during learning and memory recall processes. *Ann Neurol*. 2014;76: S24–S24.
16. Amin HU, Malik AS, Kamel N, Hussain M. A novel approach based on data redundancy for feature extraction of EEG signals. *Brain Topogr*. 2016;29(2):207–217.
17. Amin HU, Malik AS, Ahmad RF, et al. Feature extraction and classification for EEG signals using wavelet transform and machine learning techniques. *Australas Phys Eng Sci Med*. 2015;38(1):139–149.
18. Amin HU, Malik AS, Subhani AR, Badruddin N, Chooi W-T. Dynamics of scalp potential and autonomic nerve activity during intelligence test. Lee M.Hirose A, Hou Z-G, Kil R, editors. *Neural Information Processing*,Vol 8226. Heidelberg: Springer Berlin; 2013:9–16.
19. Malik AS, Khairuddin RNHR, Amin HU, et al. EEG based evaluation of stereoscopic 3D displays for viewer discomfort. *BioMed Eng OnLine*. 2015;14(1):21.

20. Amin HU, Malik AS, Mumtaz W, Badruddin N, Kamel N. Evaluation of passive polarized stereoscopic 3D display for visual & mental fatigues. *Paper presented at: Engineering in Medicine and Biology Society (EMBC), 2015 37th Annual International Conference of the IEEE*; August 25–29, 2015.
21. Amin HU, Malik AS, Badruddin N, Kamel N, Hussain M. Effects of stereoscopic 3D display technology on event-related potentials (ERPs). *Paper presented at: Neural Engineering (NER), 2015 7th International IEEE/EMBS Conference*; April 22–24, 2015.
22. Lambooij M, Fortuin M, Heynderickx I, IJsselsteijn W. Visual discomfort and visual fatigue of stereoscopic displays: a review. *J Imaging Sci Technol.* 2009;53(3) 30201-30201–30201-30214.
23. Benson AJ, CuB F. Motion sickness. *Resource Utilization and Development: A Perspective Study of Madhya Pradesh*, India; 1992:1059.
24. Ukai K, Howarth PA. Visual fatigue caused by viewing stereoscopic motion images: Background, theories, and observations. *Displays.* 2008;29(2):106–116.
25. Daugherty BC, Duchowski AT, House DH, Ramasamy C. Measuring vergence over stereoscopic video with a remote eye tracker. *Paper presented at: Proceedings of the 2010 Symposium on Eye-Tracking Research Applications*, Austin, Texas; 2010.
26. Solimini AG. Are there side effects to watching 3D movies? A prospective crossover observational study on visually induced motion sickness. *PLoS ONE.* 2013;8(2):e56160.
27. Xiao W, Fei W. A study of stereoscopic display technology and visual fatigue caused by viewing stereoscopic images. *Paper presented at: Proceedings of IEEE 2nd International Conference on Computing, Control and Industrial Engineering (CCIE)*, August 20–21, 2011.
28. Pölönen M, Järvenpää T, Bilcu B. Stereoscopic 3D entertainment and its effect on viewing comfort: Comparison of children and adults. *Appl Ergon.* 2013;44(1):151–160.
29. Reason JT, Brand JJ. *Motion Sickness.* New York: Academic Press; 1975.
30. McCauley ME. *Research Issues in Simulator Sickness: Proceedings of a Workshop.* Washington, D.C: National Academy Press; 1984.
31. Solimini AG, La Torre G, Mannocci A, Di Thiene D, Boccia A. Prevalence of symptoms of visually induced motion sickness and visual stress during and after viewing a 3D movie. *Eur J Public Health.* 2010;20:242–242.
32. Zadnik K, Mutti DO, Mitchell GL, Jones LA, Burr D, Moeschberger ML. Normal eye growth in emmetropic school children. *Optom Vis Sci.* 2004;81(11):819–828.
33. Golding JF. Motion sickness susceptibility. *Auton Neurosci Basic Clin.* 2006;129(1–2):67–76.
34. Ujike H, Watanabe H. Effects of stereoscopic presentation on visually induced motion sickness. *Paper presented at: Proceedings of SPIE—The International Society for Optical Engineering*, San Francisco, California, USA; 2011.
35. Keshavarz B, Hecht H, Zschutschke L. Intra-visual conflict in visually induced motion sickness. *Displays.* 2011;32(4):181–188.
36. Ujike H, Yokoi T, Saida S. Effects of virtual body motion on visually-induced motion sickness. *Paper presented at: Engineering in Medicine and Biology Society, 2004. IEMBS '04. 26th Annual International Conference of the IEEE*, September 1–5, 2004.

CHAPTER 11

Mobile Phone Calls

Contents

11.1 INTRODUCTION

Cellular mobile phones are an essential feature of modern telecommunications and its spread all over the world. The main function of cellular phones is to connect people for interpersonal communication. It is assumed that mobile phone users would be less lonely, more interactive with other people, and would have good psychological status. Mobile phones have different functions including calls, messages, games, access to Internet, and so on. Apart from these functions, phone calls are a direct, fast, two-way communication feature. Mobile phones establish the calls by transmitting high-frequency radio waves via their radio antennae, which convert electrical signals into radio waves and transmit them to the receiver via the base station. The range of radiated radiofrequency of mobile phones is from 450 to 2500 MHz and the radiated power from the antenna is around 125 mW and from the cell phone about 2W.[1]

Designing EEG Experiments for Studying the Brain.
DOI: http://dx.doi.org/10.1016/B978-0-12-811140-6.00011-4
© 2017 Elsevier Inc.
All rights reserved.
161

The human body may absorb some radiation and the brain of heavy users of mobile phone calls may be influenced by the electromagnetic (EM) radiation. Mobile phone users make up approximately 80% of the population in most countries, and with an increase in the quality of life-style and economic status around the world, the number of mobile users is growing. Therefore, this issue has motivated the researchers to conduct this investigation and study the effects of EM radiation on the human brain during mobile phone call use using a brain mapping technique. Various brain mapping techniques are available such as functional magnetic resonance imaging (fMRI) and electroencephalography (EEG). EEG is relatively easy to use, low cost, and has good time resolution features. EEG signals can record directly the changes occurring inside the brain in terms of voltage potentials, which can be analyzed using computational techniques to extract useful information for the assessment of brain cognitive states.[2,3] The EM radiation may modulate the EEG signals recorded over the scalp of the participants during the mobile phone calls.

In general, mobile phone users hold the mobile device very close to their right or left ear during receiving or sending phone calls and some users prolong the calls for hours; hence, the probability that human brain will absorb the EM radiation is high. Some users reported discomfort and unspecific symptoms during and after the phone calls, such as headaches and dizziness.[4] In the experiment reported in this chapter, the side effects of mobile phone calls on the human brain is investigated using EEG signals to bring awareness to the public about EM radiation, in order to take precautions during mobile phone calls.

11.2 PREVIOUS STUDIES

Previous studies have investigated the effects of mobile phones on the human brain and studied the changes in alpha frequency of EEG signals.[5] The brain signals were acquired using a call between two mobile phone devices under predefined different conditions, i.e., right ear or left ear. The results showed that alpha activity was decreased during listening to the phone call via cellular mobile phone on the right side. However, the same practice on the left side did not modulate the alpha waves and they remained stable. The reduction in alpha activity was inversely proportional to that of cell phone radiation.

Another study investigated the EM radiation for two different types of cell phones: (1) the global system for mobile communications (GSM) and

(2) code division multiple access (CDMA). The frequency and power levels of these two communications are different. The researchers conducted the experiments on 10 participants under three different conditions: (1) before using the phone, (2) using GSM, and (3) using CDMA. The brain signals were recorded and analyzed using EEG. The results suggested that in the case of GSM the power spectral density was observed to be very high and it was concluded that GSM has a greater effect on the brain signals than CDMA.[6]

Hinrikus and colleagues have investigated the effects of electromagnetic field (EMF) on the human brain using EEG. Spectral power was computed on the recorded data using linear methods and it was reported that 13–31% of the subjects were affected by the EMF, depending on the modulation frequency.[7]

Mann et al. examined the effects of EMF on brain signals during sleep. Twelve volunteers participated in the experiments, which were composed of five stages of sleep at night and during exposure to radiofrequency (RF) emissions from a mobile phone. EEG signals were recorded and analyzed; the findings indicated that spectral power during REM sleep was increased by 5% during EMF exposure; however, no changes were reported in other sleep stages.[8]

Reiser and Dimpfel studied the effects of mobile phone radiation on the brain. They employed 36 participants and studied under three experimental conditions: before, during, and after the call. The findings suggested that relative alpha power during and after exposure is increased.[9]

In addition, Trueman et al. studied the effect of mobile phone EMF emissions on the brain using EEG signals. In their experiment, 10 volunteers participated during the presence and absence of RF. The RF was generated using two mobile technologies. In the first condition, the RF was generated by GSM phone with disabled speaker and modified to full radiation power transmission. In the second condition, the RF emissions were generated by a nonmodified GSM mobile phone in active standby mode. The participants were studied in each condition for minutes. The statistical analysis unfolded the findings, indicating a difference in the full-power mode condition within the EEG alpha (8–13 Hz) and beta (13–32 Hz) bands.[10]

Besides, it is common practice, especially for teenagers, to use mobile devices as a replacement for alarm clocks underneath the pillow during sleep. This investigation raises concern about this practice.

11.3 IMPORTANCE OF STUDYING THE EFFECTS OF MOBILE PHONE CALLS

The cellular or mobile phone is one of the great inventions of the 20th century. In the first decade of the 21st century, there has been a cellular phone craze among the young generation due to the powerful features of display technology, besides use for making phone calls. The key features of mobile phone technology, including text messages, email, calls, Internet searching, videos, games, social networking, and social applications, have such widespread interest that the young generation is fully addicted.

Presently, the mobile phone provides an incredible array of functions, such as huge storage for personal contact directories, pictures, movies, GPS tracking, TV streaming, and so on. The basic working principle of the cellular phone is that it converts voice or text information into an electrical signal, which is then transmitted as radio waves (a kind of electromagnetic or EM wave) to the destination device via the intermediate base station. The mobile phone devices are continuously active and ready for transmitting and receiving EM waves. The effects of EM radiation on brain health are reported in previous research as a serious risk factor.[11–14] The users' feedback indicated that phone calls cause fatigue and dizziness[13]; while long-term users are more vulnerable to brain tumors.[15,16] The reason may be that EM waves penetrate into the brain,[17–19] especially the auditory regions in the temporal lobe, because mobile phone users keep the device very close to their ears when receiving calls. Thus, the most affected regions of the brain are the auditory regions in the temporal lobe. The temporal lobe is also functional in memory tasks; thus, EM radiation alters neuronal activities during memory tasks.[20]

Neuroimaging techniques such as EEG have been used to study the effects of cellular phones on the human brain, e.g., in memory tasks and during resting states.[20,21] Since the practice of keeping mobile phones set close to the ear is common, it will be interesting to investigate the use of mobile phones both in conditions of very close to the ear (in other words, close to the brain) and at a distance while receiving a phone call. In addition, using the left ear or right ear (left or right of the brain) during receiving phone calls will explore the brain regions most vulnerable to EM radiation.

11.4 PROBLEM DESCRIPTION

Cellular phone technology works by transmitting signals through EM waves to produce very high radio frequencies. The human brain absorbs

EM waves during phone calls, causing health problems, particularly near the regions of the ear where mobile devices are normally held during usage. Evidence about the issues of mobile call usage is from users who have reported headaches and dizziness during and/or after phone calls. Such reasons motivated the researchers to investigate and monitor any potential risk of mobile phones on public health. Although the scientific literature on this issue is vast and apparently indicates widely varying effects across studies, this study was conducted to explore the effects of mobile phone calls on the brain using a direct measurement technique of the human brain.

The experiment had the following two main objectives:

- To explore and study the effects of EM radiation during mobile phone calls on the human brain using EEG signals.
- To explore ways to minimize the effects of direct radiation from the mobile phone on the human brain.

11.5 SOFTWARE AND HARDWARE

A description of the equipment and software used in this experiment is provided in Table 11.1.

11.6 EXPERIMENT DESIGN AND PROTOCOL

11.6.1 Target Population

In this study, the students on the university campus were the target population. All the students on the university campus were the entire set of units for which the findings of the research had been generalized. Three levels of students were studying on the campus at the time of experiment, i.e., foundation level, undergraduate, and postgraduate level. Equal opportunity was given to all students who met the inclusion criteria to become a participant.

11.6.2 Inclusion Criteria

- Participant must be a student in Universiti Teknologi PETRONAS
- Participant should be between 18 and 25 years of age
- Participant must be physically and mentally healthy

11.6.3 Exclusion Criteria

- Unable to provide written consent (Appendix 2C)
- Failed to meet the requirements mentioned in the inclusion criteria

Table 11.1 Description of hardware (equipment) and software

S. No.	Equipment	Description
01	Emotiv EPOC headset	14 EEG channel plus 2 reference system offer optional positioning for accurate spatial resolution.
02	Re-nu multipurpose solution	A few drops of this multipurpose saline solution to saturate the white hydrator pad.
03	Emotiv EPOC hydrator pack	16 fully assembled felt-based sensor assemblies with gold-plated contacts.
04	Emotiv Insight charging cable	Replacement charging cable for the Insight headset.
05	USB receiver	Replacement USB receiver for Emotiv EPOC, EPOC+, and Insight neuroheadsets.
06	Mobile cell phone	A Nokia C3 mobile set is used in this experiment.
07	EEGLAB	EEGLAB tool is used for artifact removal.
08	Neuroguide 2.6.1	Neuroguide is used for absolute power and coherence analysis. Details on Neuroguide have been provided in previous chapters.
09	MATLAB	MATLAB R2010a is used for analysis. Details on MATLAB are provided in previous chapters.

11.6.4 Sample Size Calculation

The sample size computation for this study was not predefined, as it was a pilot study. Further research on this topic may be required to properly compute the sample size using the mean differences among the different conditions (i.e., left and right side, with distance and without distance) of this study, which are reported in the published papers.

11.6.5 Participant Recruitment

Twenty-seven healthy participants were recruited from students of Universiti Teknologi PETRONAS to participate in the study, including male, female, and different nationalities. All the participants were free from any medication, skin allergy, or head injury. Participants suffering from headaches were excluded from the study because this may affect the behavior of the EEG signals. Furthermore, only right-handed participants were recruited because the participants were required to hold the mobile device in hand, so using the right or left hand may affect the brain functions. Therefore, all participants recruited were of the same handedness.

11.6.6 Experiment Design

The experiment consisted of a total of six conditions. Two conditions were used for baseline EEG recordings, i.e., EEG recording before and EEG recording after the mobile usage. The four other conditions were used during listening to a mobile phone call, including two conditions for the right side and two conditions for the left side. Each side (right or left) included two EEG measurements. One measurement was taken when the participant was using the mobile phone very close to his/her ear (touching the ear) while another measurement was taken while the mobile phone was kept 2 cm away from the ear during listening to the phone call. The final measurement was taken after mobile phone usage to measure the brain signals and to detect whether headache or dizziness was experienced after the calls. The EEG measurements were recorded using Emotiv EPOC 16 electrodes, as shown in Fig. 11.1, connected to a PC to show the brain signals.

11.6.7 Experiment Procedure

Each participant was briefed about the experiment and asked to read the informed consent form and subject information. In case of any ambiguity, they were encouraged to clarify with the experimenter. After signing the

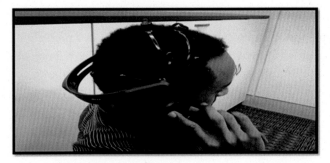

Figure 11.1 Emotiv EPOC 16 electrodes.

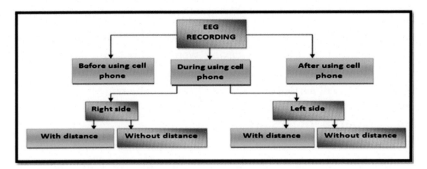

Figure 11.2 Block diagram of experiment protocol.

consent form, each participant was asked to fill out a questionnaire (see Appendix 11A) to record the history of the participant and the information on mobile phone usage. After filling out the questionnaire, the participant was asked to sit in a relaxed mode in the EEG recording room. The Emotiv EEG kit was prepared and set on the participant's head per the recommended procedure. The measurements of EEG were recorded for the effect of cell phone use using EEG under six conditions, i.e., before using the cell phone, during the use of the cell phone (4 subconditions), and after using the cell phone; please refer to Fig. 11.2.

The duration of each session was 5 minutes long, and between sessions, participants were given a few minutes for rest. The participants were instructed to remain silent during all the sessions to minimize the artifacts in EEG recordings. The experiment was completed in approximately 1 hour.

Table 11.2 EEG data description

S. No.	File name	EEG description
01	A_1.edf	Five minutes EEG recording before using the mobile phone in rest condition.
02	B_1.edf	Five minutes EEG recorded during phone call at right side without distance.
03	C_1.edf	Five minutes EEG recorded during phone call at right side with distance. The distance is 2 cm.
04	D_1.edf	Five minutes EEG recorded during phone call at left side without distance.
05	E_1.edf	Five minutes EEG recorded during phone call at left side with distance. The distance is 2 cm.
06	F_1.edf	Five minutes EEG recording after completing all the sessions with phone calls. This recording was performed in rest condition.

11.7 DATA DESCRIPTION

EEG raw and clean data for one participant is provided with this book. The details of these files are provided in Table 11.2. To access these files, please go to the directory BookData\Chap11\EEG in the data files accompanying this book. For the complete dataset of 27 participants, please contact the authors at brainexpbook@gmail.com.

ACKNOWLEDGMENTS

This chapter provides the details of the experiment design reported in the BE FYP report of Eithar Isameldin Ahmed Nouri, which is available at Universiti Teknologi PETRONAS.

REFERENCES

1. Sage C, Carpenter DO. Public health implications of wireless technologies. *Pathophysiology.* 2009;16(2):233–246.
2. Amin HU, Malik AS, Ahmad RF, et al. Feature extraction and classification for EEG signals using wavelet transform and machine learning techniques. *Australas Phys Eng Sci Med.* 2015;38(1):139–149.
3. Amin HU, Malik AS, Kamel N, Hussain M. A novel approach based on data redundancy for feature extraction of EEG signals. *Brain Topogr.* 2016;29(2):207–217.
4. Röösli M. Radiofrequency electromagnetic field exposure and non-specific symptoms of ill health: a systematic review. *Environ Res.* 2008;107(2):277–287.
5. Murat ZH, AbdulKadir RSS, Isa RM, Taib MN. The effects of mobile phone usage on human brainwave using EEG. *Paper presented at: Computer Modelling and Simulation (UKSim), 2011 UkSim 13th International Conference;* 2011.

6. Tyagi A, Duhan M, Bhatia D. Effect of mobile phone radiation on brain activity–GSM Vs CDMA. *Int J Sci Technol Manag.* 2011;2(2):1–5.
7. Hinrikus H, Bachmann M, Lass J, Karai D, Tuulik V. Effect of low frequency modulated microwave exposure on human EEG: individual sensitivity. *Bioelectromagnetics.* 2008;29(7):527–538.
8. Mann K, Röschke J. Effects of pulsed high-frequency electromagnetic fields on human sleep. *Neuropsychobiology.* 1996;33(1):41–47.
9. Reiser H, Dimpfel W, Schober F. The influence of electromagnetic fields on human brain activity. *Eur J Med Res.* 1995;1(1):27–32.
10. Trueman G, Tang L, Abdel-Rahman U, Abdel-Rahman W, Ong K, Cosic I. Human brain wave activity during exposure to radiofrequency field emissions from mobile phones. *Australas Phys Eng Sci Med.* 2003;26(4):162–167.
11. Seitz H, Stinner D, Eikmann T, Herr C, Röösli M. Electromagnetic hypersensitivity (EHS) and subjective health complaints associated with electromagnetic fields of mobile phone communication—a literature review published between 2000 and 2004. *Sci Total Environ.* 2005;349(1–3):45–55.
12. Hossmann KA, Hermann D. Effects of electromagnetic radiation of mobile phones on the central nervous system. *Bioelectromagnetics.* 2003;24(1):49–62.
13. Al-Khlaiwi T, Meo SA. Association of mobile phone radiation with fatigue, headache, dizziness, tension and sleep disturbance in Saudi population. *Saudi Med J.* 2004;25(6):732–736.
14. Lönn S, Ahlbom A, Hall P, Feychting M. Mobile phone use and the risk of acoustic neuroma. *Epidemiology.* 2004;15(6):653–659.
15. Lönn S, Ahlbom A, Hall P, Feychting M, Group SIS. Long-term mobile phone use and brain tumor risk. *Am J Epidemiol.* 2005;161(6):526–535.
16. Inskip PD, Tarone RE, Hatch EE, et al. Cellular-telephone use and brain tumors. *N Engl J Med.* 2001;344(2):79–86.
17. Schüz J, Steding-Jessen M, Hansen S, et al. Long-term mobile phone use and the risk of vestibular schwannoma: a Danish nationwide cohort study. *Am J Epidemiol.* 2011;174(4):416–422.
18. Kesari KK, Siddiqui MH, Meena R, Verma H, Kumar S. Cell phone radiation exposure on brain and associated biological systems. *Indian J Exp Biol.* 2013;51(3):187–200.
19. Khurana VG, Teo C, Kundi M, Hardell L, Carlberg M. Cell phones and brain tumors: a review including the long-term epidemiologic data. *Surg Neurol.* 2009;72(3):205–214.
20. Krause CM, Sillanmäki L, Koivisto M, et al. Effects of electromagnetic field emitted by cellular phones on the EEG during a memory task. *Neuroreport.* 2000;11(4):761–764.
21. Curcio G, Ferrara M, Moroni F, D'inzeo G, Bertini M, De Gennaro L. Is the brain influenced by a phone call? an EEG study of resting wakefulness. *Neurosci Res.* 2005;53(3):265–270.

CHAPTER 12

Drivers' Cognitive Distraction

Contents

12.1 INTRODUCTION

Driving is a complex task that requires motor and visual capabilities along with high alertness, mental planning, and memory resources. Individual differences exist corresponding to these cognitive capabilities, which are natural in human beings. In addition to individual differences, there are also other sources, such as drugs and alcohol, which significantly increase driver distraction and cause 20–80% of crashes.[1] More seriously, inattention was found to be the largest factor behind all crashes and near crashes (78%), reported by Dingus et al. in a study of 100 car accidents.[2]

A situation during driving operation in which the driver's attention turns away from driving toward a competing activity such as attending a cell phone call, using the navigation system and audio system, absentmindedness, daydreaming, and decision making, is known as *driving distraction*. These competing activities have been reported as factors in driver distraction and traffic accidents (see Ref. [3] for review). Driver distraction can be of two major types: visual distraction and cognitive distraction. The

Designing EEG Experiments for Studying the Brain.
DOI: http://dx.doi.org/10.1016/B978-0-12-811140-6.00012-6
© 2017 Elsevier Inc.
All rights reserved.

former (*visual distraction*) is the state where the driver's eye focus is away from the track and the latter (*cognitive distraction*) is absentmindedness or attention deviation from the driving operation. Both of these distractions impair driving safety and affect the driver's performance. The negative effects of cognitive distraction on visual information processing during driving have been reported by many previous studies.[4–6]

The focus of the experiment reported in this chapter is on drivers' cognitive distraction. To understand drivers' psychological behavior and sources of distraction, the electroencephalography (EEG) technique was employed. EEG signals help to study the neuronal changes occurring due to distraction during driving operation. EEG signals directly measure the neuronal changes occurring due to any distraction including driving distraction and can be quantitatively analyzed using computational techniques to determine useful information for assessment of brain distraction.[7,8] Also, the psychological behavior can be better understood in real time during driving operation. Hence, in this study, the participants were investigated in both cognitive state and noncognitive state, in order to compare the changes occurring in EEG signals due to cognitive distraction. The following two objectives were defined for this experiment:

- To study the effects of cognitive distraction on drivers' behavior and driving performance using EEG signals.
- To identify the specific brain regions and certain brain oscillations involved in driving operation as well as cognitive activities.

12.2 IMPORTANCE OF STUDYING DRIVER DISTRACTION

Driving is an essential activity in our daily lives. Every day, we trudge through traffic to take children to school and pick them up from school, as well as to get to work; we use highways to get across town and haul tons of goods and commodities on trucks to run our businesses. It is such a widespread activity that everyone of us is directly or indirectly affected by drivers' actions. To be safe, drivers need their full attention on the road and should be alert at all times in order to react to potential life-threatening situations. Basic driver needs, including sufficient sleep, good physical and mental health, and good training in driving principles, are no longer enough in the modern technological era. The reason is that with the advent of technologies involving automobiles and communication, e.g., mobile phone technology, there is increased probability of accidents, which is a huge risk for both drivers and passengers' lives.

The automobile industry has introduced LCD screens in cars, which is an improvement in the manufacturing of vehicles and entertainment for the passengers, who can watch videos and movies in order to be relaxed and not bored. However, LCD screens increase the risks of attentional diversion and visual distraction for the drivers, as proven by research evidence.[9–13] In addition, with advancements in communication with the advent of mobile phones and smart phones, it has become a necessity for everyone to keep their mobile phone device active. Mobile phones have many interesting features, some of which are either necessary to be used while driving, or someone may be addicted enough to use them even while driving. Research has proven that during driving, the use of mobile phones in any capacity, either texting or calling, causes distraction visually and mentally for the drivers.[14–19] Such inattentional and visually distracted moments cause serious casualties and accidents. The effects of visual and cognitive load distraction have been studied in previous research[4,20,21]; however, previous studies focused on behavioral investigations rather than objective or quantitative assessment.[3,22] Behavioral assessments such as collecting drivers' feedback after operating a driver simulator in an experimental environment or counting the number of mistakes during operating the simulator could not explain the actual changes in the brain neuronal activities that cause the behavior of the drivers due to visual or cognitive distractions. Therefore, the drivers' distraction is currently being investigated with neuroimaging techniques such as EEG.

The EEG technique can be easily used in the experimental environment along with the driver simulator for long duration and can record the neuronal changes associated with driving skill, attention, visual distraction, and cognitive distraction. The researchers may find a real time monitoring solution for drivers with the use of EEG. Since there are many open questions, such as how EEG sensors can be placed on the drivers' head in real time during driving on highways, and how flexible, portable, and how much of a distraction the EEG sensors will be for the drivers, this EEG research is still in the development stage in drivers' safety as well as in the automobile industry. However, the EEG technique explores the neuronal changes of the drivers induced due to visual and cognitive distractions as well as attentional diversion.

12.3 SOFTWARE AND HARDWARE

The equipment and software used in this study is described in Table 12.1.

Table 12.1 Description of hardware and software

S. No.	Equipment	Description
01	EGI EEG 300 Amp	This EEG system provides a dense array EEG acquisition with high resolution for research and clinical applications. The manufacturer, EGI, has designed the Clinical Geodesic EEG System (GES) 300 for better treatment and care of patients.
02	EGI EEG 128 channels nets	The 128-channel EGI nets are available in different sizes to fit on the participant's head and record EEG signals.
03	Control III	Control III disinfectant cleaning solution is a concentrated disinfectant and is recommended by the manufacturer for cleaning of EEG caps and electrodes.
04	Potassium chloride	For standard 2-hour recordings, potassium chloride solution is used for rapid application. The potassium chloride is in powder form and can be mixed with distilled water.
05	City Car Driving 2.4.4	City Car Driving is a new car simulator, developed to help users experience car driving in different conditions and in different big cities.
06	LG display, 42-inch	The LG 42-inch display was used with the City Car Driving simulator to display the driving environment.
07	Net Station 4.2	EGI's Net Station is an integrated software package for EEG acquisition, review, and analysis.
08	MATLAB	MATLAB is used for analysis of EEG data. The description of MATLAB is provided in previous chapters (see Chapter 7: 2D and 3D Educational Contents).

12.4 EXPERIMENT DESIGN AND PROTOCOL

12.4.1 Target Population

In this experiment, the students on the university campus were the target population. All the students on the university campus were the entire set of units for which the findings of the research had been generalized. Equal opportunity was given to all the students who met the inclusion criteria to become a participant.

12.4.2 Inclusion Criteria

- Participants should have be between 18 and 24 years of age.
- Participants must be physically and mentally healthy.

12.4.3 Exclusion Criteria

The exclusion criteria are the requirements used for exclusion of participants from this study. The participants were excluded in this study when they failed to meet the requirements in the inclusion criteria.

12.4.4 Sample Size Calculation

This was a pilot study and the number of participants in the experiment was based on expert opinion. Further studies may use the results of this experimentation to statistically compute the exact sample size and generalize the results of this study. For the results of this experiment, please see the published papers listed in Section 12.6.

12.4.5 Participant Recruitment

In this experiment, 42 healthy volunteers aged between 18 and 24 years (mean: 21.76 and SD: 1.65) including 33 males and 9 females were recruited. All the recruited participants had normal or corrected to normal vision ability and had no history of brain disorders. The participants were allowed to practice the driving simulator for approximately 10 minutes because they had no previous experience operating the driving simulator. Further, the participants were allowed to stop their participation in the experiment at any time without any penalty if they were not feeling comfortable.

12.4.6 Experiment Design

In the experiment, the participants were exposed to two type of tasks: primary and secondary tasks.

12.4.6.1 Driving (Primary Task)

This task required driving for 30 minutes duration and paying full attention to all the driving rules, such as driving 80 km/hour speed, and using indicator lights to turn left/light or when needed. During the driving task, the driving environment was limited to one simulator vehicle on a highway road in order to provide same conditions to all the participants. This task was used both in session 1 and session 2. Session 1 was used as the control session, because the participants just performed the driving operation without any distraction; while session 2 consisted of the driving task along with cognitive distraction. The cognitive distraction is referred to as a secondary task. Each of the sessions was 30 minutes long.

12.4.6.2 Cognitive Task (Secondary Task)

The cognitive task consisted of logical questions requiring mental decision making and mathematical calculation to use the cognitive resources of the participant during the driving task. As a result, cognitive distraction was induced by involving participants in other activities (see example questions used in this experiment in Table 12.2). The second session (driving distraction session) was segmented into six consecutive intervals of "attentive" and "distractive" driving as shown in Fig. 12.1. In the distractive segment of driving, the participants were asked logical questions and they were instructed to answer accurately. While the questions were being asked, they were instructed to listen to the question and stay calm with minimum movement and pay attention to the road and driving and

Table 12.2 Example of logical problems in the cognitive task

Problem	Response
Odometer is to mileage as compass is to: A. speed B. hiking C. needle D. direction	D
Elated is to despondent as enlightened is to: A. aware B. ignorant C. miserable D. tolerant	B
Careful is to cautious as boastful is to: A. arrogant B. humble C. joyful D. suspicious	A
Pride is to lion as shoal is to: A. teacher B. student C. self-respect D. fish	D
I want to make 12 cakes. If I know that 6 kg of flour is enough for 36 cakes, how much flour will I need?	2 kg
When a bucket is full it holds exactly 1/2 L. A jug holds 500 mL. How many full jugs of water will I need to fill the bucket?	1 jug
Find the cost of 4.5 kg of sugar at 20 p per 500 g.	180 p

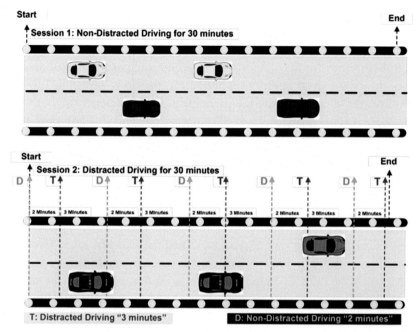

Figure 12.1 Experimental design.[23] The first row indicates the driving with distraction and second row indicates the driving without distraction.

think about the answer silently. The duration of the distractive segment was 3 minutes and the attentive segment was 2 minutes.

12.4.7 Experiment Procedure

This experiment consisted of two sessions. In the first session, when a participant arrives at the experiment room, he/she is briefed about the experiment and asked to practice driving in the driving simulator for almost 10 minutes before setting the EEG cap for data recording. The driving simulator was a simple device and consisted of steering, foot pedals, and gear lever along with a virtual reality-based highway driving environment. During the experimental tasks, the driving surroundings were restricted to only one simulator vehicle on road, using identical cars—Toyota Corolla with automatic gear system—and with medium traffic. A display screen was used at distance of 1 m from the participant at the same level of the steering wheel.

After practicing the driving, each participant was asked to perform the experimental task, in which EEG data was recorded. Participants were trained to drive for 30 minutes and concentrate on driving rules as per instructions given. In the second session, the participants were instructed to do the driving task the same as in the first session, but they had to carefully listen to the secondary task, in which the participants needed to respond to the logical questions. The logical questions were asked by the experimenter standing beside the participant. In the experiment, both sessions were counterbalanced, i.e., half of the participants first completed the control session (session 1) and then the second session, while the other half started with the driving distraction session (session 2) and then completed the control session.

12.5 EEG DATA DESCRIPTION

The EEG was recorded via 128 scalp loci using the EGI HydroCel Geodesic Sensor Net with Amps 300 amplifier (Electrical Geodesic Inc., Eugene, OR, USA) for all the tasks. The electrode Cz was used as a reference for all 128 electrodes. Impedance was maintained below 5 KΩ and the sampling rate was 500 samples per second. The sampling rate of raw EEG data was 500 while the clean data was downsampled to 250 points per second.

12.5.1 Experiment Data Accompanying This Book

EEG raw data and clean data files for one-subject are provided with this book. The details of these files are provided in Table 12.3. To access these files, please go to the directory BookData\Chapter12 in the data files

Table 12.3 EEG data files with description

S. No.	File name	Description
01	Sub1_c1_raw.mat	This is EEG one-subject raw data recorded during session 1 while driving the simulator without any distraction. The data file contains 128 channels with Cz as a reference and sampling rate is 500 points per second.
02	Sub1_c2_raw.mat	This is EEG one-subject raw data recorded during session 2 while driving the simulator along with cognitive distraction, i.e., answering the logical questions during operating the driving simulator. The data properties are the same as recorded in session 1.
03	Sub1_c1_clean.mat	This is the clean EEG form of the data file described in serial number 01 in this table.
04	Sub1_c2_clean.mat	This is the clean EEG form of the data file described in serial number 02 in this table.

accompanying this book. For the complete dataset of 42 participants, please contact the authors at brainexpbook@gmail.com.

12.6 RELEVANT PAPERS

This section provides a list of some of the papers that have utilized the data acquired from the experiment described in this chapter. The following papers should be cited when using the experiment design or the data provided with this chapter.

1. Almahasneh H, Chooi W-T, Kamel N, Malik AS. Deep in thought while driving: an EEG study on drivers' cognitive distraction. *Transp Res Part F Traffic Psychol Behav.* 2014;26:218–226.
2. Almahasneh H, Kamel N, Walter N, Malik AS. r-principal subspace for driver cognitive state classification. In: *Engineering in Medicine and Biology Society (EMBC), 2015 37th Annual International Conference of the IEEE;* 2015, pp. 4118–4121.

ACKNOWLEDGMENTS

This chapter provides the details of the experiment design available in the papers mentioned in Section 12.5 and in the PhD thesis of Mr. Hossam Almahasneh, which is available at Universiti Teknologi PETRONAS.

REFERENCES

1. Stutts JC, Association AA. *The Role of Driver Distraction in Traffic Crashes.* Washington, DC: AAA Foundation for Traffic Safety; 2001.
2. Dingus TA, Klauer S, Neale V, et al. The 100-car naturalistic driving study, Phase II-results of the 100-car field experiment; 2006.
3. Young K, Regan M, Hammer M. Driver distraction: a review of the literature. *Distracted Driv.* 2007:379–405.
4. Engström J, Johansson E, Östlund J. Effects of visual and cognitive load in real and simulated motorway driving. *Transp Res Part F Traffic Psychol Behav.* 2005;8(2):97–120.
5. Strayer DL, Cooper JM, Turrill J, Coleman J, Medeiros-Ward N, Biondi F. Measuring cognitive distraction in the automobile; 2013.
6. Harbluk JL, Noy YI, Eizenman M. The impact of cognitive distraction on driver visual behaviour and vehicle control; 2002.
7. Amin HU, Malik AS, Kamel N, Hussain M. A novel approach based on data redundancy for feature extraction of EEG signals. *Brain Topogr.* 2016;29(2):207–217.
8. Amin HU, Malik AS, Ahmad RF, et al. Feature extraction and classification for EEG signals using wavelet transform and machine learning techniques. *Australas Phys Eng Sci Med.* 2015;38(1):139–149.
9. Knoll PM. The use of displays in automotive applications. *J Soc Inf Disp.* 1997;5(3):165–172.
10. White C, Fern L, Caird J, et al. The Effects of Dvd Modality on Drivers' performance. *Paper presented at: Proceedings of the 37th Annual Conference of the Association of Canadian Ergonomists;* 2006.

11. Stavrinos D, Jones JL, Garner AA, et al. Impact of distracted driving on safety and traffic flow. *Accid Anal Prev.* 2013;61:63–70.
12. Sumiła M. Evaluation of the drivers' distraction caused by dashboard MMI interface. *Paper presented at: International Conference on Transport Systems Telematics*; 2014.
13. Pfleging B, Schneegass S, Schmidt A. Multimodal interaction in the car: combining speech and gestures on the steering wheel. *Paper presented at: Proceedings of the 4th International Conference on Automotive User Interfaces and Interactive Vehicular Applications*; 2012.
14. Redelmeier DA, Tibshirani RJ. Association between cellular-telephone calls and motor vehicle collisions. *N Engl J Med.* 1997;336(7):453–458.
15. Wilson FA, Stimpson JP. Trends in fatalities from distracted driving in the United States, 1999 to 2008. *Am J Public Health.* 2010;100(11):2213–2219.
16. Nelson E, Atchley P, Little TD. The effects of perception of risk and importance of answering and initiating a cellular phone call while driving. *Accid Anal Prev.* 2009;41(3):438–444.
17. Klauer SG, Guo F, Simons-Morton BG, Ouimet MC, Lee SE, Dingus TA. Distracted driving and risk of road crashes among novice and experienced drivers. *N Engl J Med.* 2014;370(1):54–59.
18. Nemme HE, White KM. Texting while driving: Psychosocial influences on young people's texting intentions and behaviour. *Accid Anal Prev.* 2010;42(4):1257–1265.
19. Farmer CM, Braitman KA, Lund AK. Cell phone use while driving and attributable crash risk. *Traffic Inj Prev.* 2010;11(5):466–470.
20. Petridou E, Moustaki M. Human factors in the causation of road traffic crashes. *Eur J Epidemiol.* 2000;16(9):819–826.
21. Perrow C. *Normal Accidents: Living with High Risk Technologies.* Princeton, NJ: Princeton University Press; 2011.
22. Rudin-Brown CM, Parker HA. Behavioural adaptation to adaptive cruise control (ACC): implications for preventive strategies. *Transp Res Part F Traffic Psychol Behav.* 2004;7(2):59–76.
23. Almahasneh H, Chooi W-T, Kamel N, Malik AS. Deep in thought while driving: An EEG study on drivers' cognitive distraction. *Transp Res Part F Traffic Psychol Behav.* 2014;26:218–226.

CHAPTER 13

Drivers' Drowsiness

Contents

13.1 INTRODUCTION

Driving is a complex task that needs physical resources as well as mental alertness. The requirement of full mental alertness makes it a riskier task because humans have limited capability to be attentive for long amounts of time. Lack of attention, absentmindedness, and/or drowsiness can cause serious major injuries and loss of life for travelers including drivers and passengers. There are many factors involved in road accidents such as weather, road condition, vehicle condition, drivers' distraction, drivers' driving skills and drowsiness. The state of drowsiness is often referred to as sleepiness, which means that the driver/person has a tendency to fall asleep.

The sleep cycle of humans is divided into three categories: wakefulness, nonrapid eye movement (NREM), and rapid eye movement (REM).[1] Wakefulness is the state of consciousness and completely being alert, in which a person can perform physical and mental tasks without any inattention. The NREM state is further divided into three stages.

Designing EEG Experiments for Studying the Brain.
DOI: http://dx.doi.org/10.1016/B978-0-12-811140-6.00013-8
© 2017 Elsevier Inc.
All rights reserved.

Stage one is related to drowsiness while stages two and three are associated with light sleep and deep sleep states, respectively. The REM state is characterized by quick and random movement of the eyes and muscles. Drowsiness is an intermediate state between sleepiness and being awake. In the state of drowsiness, an individual's attention and vigilance toward the tasks are reduced.[2] In driving operation, drowsiness is very hazardous and risky, where the driver's loss of attention and increased response time can cause road accidents resulting in serious injuries and deaths. This usually occurs when the driver is extremely drowsy, unaware of his or her surroundings, and fails to make the right decisions prior to a crash.

Recent studies reported that drowsiness at the wheel is one of the major contributing factors of road accidents, causing a large number of deaths, serious injuries, and financial losses. Drowsy driving accidents mostly occur between midnight and 6:00 a.m., or in the late afternoon (during both times, there are dips in circadian rhythm, the internal body clock that regulates sleep). The US National Highway Traffic Safety Administration (NHTSA) reported that there were 846 fatalities due to drowsiness in 2014, which constitutes 2.6% of all fatalities. Further, between 2005 and 2009 there was an estimated average of 83,000 crashes each year related to drowsy driving (see Fig. 13.1[3]). The statistics include 886 fatal crashes, an estimated 37,000 injury crashes, and around 45,000 incidents of property damage.

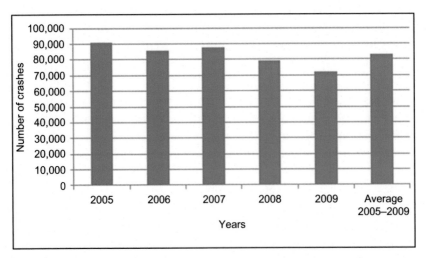

Figure 13.1 NHTSA statistics on crashes caused by driver drowsiness from 2005 to 2009.

The research investigation of Centre for Accident Research and Road Safety (CARRS) in Queensland, Australia shows that fatigue or drowsiness is one of the contributing factors toward road accidents apart from other factors, such as speeding and drinking alcohol. In fact, 20–30% of all deaths on the road are the direct result of drowsiness.[4] The statistics also show that the risk of death in road accidents is 13.5 times higher in rural areas than in urban areas. The possibility of such crashes is more likely on long straight roads, which definitely highlights the risk that drowsiness poses. The reports also indicate that many other crashes are not verified by the police, suggesting accidents due to drowsiness can be much higher in number and have been underestimated in the past.

In Malaysia, traffic accidents involving public transport and private cars are also a serious problem. A survey report by the Malaysian Institute of Road Safety (MIROS) shows that the rate of road accidents in Malaysia is larger in number as compared to other countries.[5] Traffic statistics show that the total number of accidents from 1997 to 2007 has increased from 215,632 to 363,314 and one of the major contributing factors is driver drowsiness.[5] The report also indicates that a 58% increase in fatal accidents has been observed from 2006 to 2007 and these fatalities occur due to crashes involving buses. These crashes are quite large in number and if not resolved, they may increase in upcoming years.

Preventing accidents from happening due to drowsiness at the wheel has been an area of extensive research in the past few years. Researchers are taking keen interest to develop systems that can detect driver drowsiness and alert the driver before the crash. The importance of such a system can be easily understood as it might be able to decrease the amount of road accidents caused by drivers' drowsiness to a great extent.

13.2 IMPORTANCE OF STUDYING DRIVERS' DROWSINESS

Driver drowsiness is one of the main causes of road accidents. It is a serious hazard in transportation systems for drivers' safety. There are various symptoms that indicate to the drivers to stop driving and take a rest; e.g., heavy eyelids, difficulty in focusing, missing traffic signs, yawning, trouble keeping the head up, feeling restless and irritable, drifting from lane, blurry vision, rubbing eyes, etc. However, avoiding these signs could lead to a serious or fatal accident while driving.[6] It has been reported that sleep-related casualties are a major issue in the transport system[7,8] as well as for the automobile industry.

Different drivers' drowsiness detection metrics have been proposed in the literature that have focused on lane deviations, high level of fatigue, video-based system (detecting eyes closing or eye blinks).[9–12] The reported methods in the literature are based on various measurements including subjective measure, vehicle-based measure, behavior measure, and physiological measure. However, no perfect alert system for drivers' drowsiness detection exists, so each proposed system has limitations in terms of cost, effectiveness, flexibility, or practical implementation.

The use of neuroimaging techniques such as EEG can help the researchers to test for drowsy drivers in a simulated experimental environment, since it is not safe or ethical to allow a drowsy driver on the road for an experiment. Thus, the simulated environment helps the researchers to control the costs, efficiency, safety, and easy-to-collect data. In addition, the use of EEG signals can record the specific pattern that changes with the sleepy state or loss of alertness. Therefore, in future an EEG-based alert system may be introduced by the automobile companies for informing the drowsy drivers either by sound alarm or direct controlling of the vehicle.

13.3 PROBLEM STATEMENT

Driving is one of the most common activities in daily life. There are more vehicles on the road than ever and this number continues to increase with the passage of time due to improvement in people's lifestyles. Vehicle manufacturing companies are trying to increase safety systems in the new models, but these efforts are still not enough to decrease vehicle-related accidents, which keep on increasing due to human factors. As stated earlier, driver drowsiness is the major contributor to road accidents. Therefore, it is necessary to examine the changes that occur in the human physiological state from alert to drowsy states. It is hypothesized from this study that driver drowsiness affects the human physiological state and shows variations in brain signals.

The work presented in this chapter focuses on the detection of driver drowsiness by utilizing the quantitative features of electroencephalogram (EEG) and electrocardiogram (ECG) signals. EEG signals directly measure the neuronal changes occurring due to drowsiness or cognitive fatigue and can be quantitatively analyzed using computational techniques to determine useful information for assessment of brain states.[13,14] Similarly, ECG signals that refer to the dynamics of heartbeats are useful to study the heart rate variability (HRV) during any mental state such as drowsiness.[15] These signals are recorded in a simulator-based driving environment in which subjects

Table 13.1 Description of hardware and software

S. No.	Equipment	Description
01	Driving simulator	Driving simulator is used to create driving environment in experimental room.
02	Enobio Star Stim EEG 20 channels	Enobio wireless electrophysiology sensor system is a wearable EEG device, which is good for medium density recording for research applications.
03	ECG electrode	Enobio provides additional electrodes along with EEG sensors to record the heartbeats.
04	Cameras	Four different camera views are recorded during experimentation using webcam and video cameras.
05	Sony 40-inch TV screen	TV screen is used to display the driving environment for the experiment.

were allowed to drive in a monotonous driving environment so that they experience drowsiness. The following were the objectives of the study:

- To detect the transition from alert to drowsy state using physiological signals.
- To investigate and identify significant features in EEG and ECG signals for the detection of driver drowsiness.

13.4 SOFTWARE AND HARDWARE

A description of the equipment and software used in this experiment is provided in Table 13.1.

13.5 EXPERIMENT DESIGN AND PROTOCOL

13.5.1 Target Population

In this study, the students on the university campus were the target population. All the students on the university campus were the entire set of units for which the findings of the research had been generalized. The participants who were interested in taking part in the experiment were shortlisted based upon the following inclusion and exclusion criteria.

13.5.2 Inclusion Criteria

- Participant must have a driving experience of at least 2 years to be eligible in the study.
- Participant must have a valid driving license.
- Participant must have no serious injuries or mental disorders such as epilepsy, migraine, seizures, or tumor.
- Participant must not be under any medication that might disturb the physiological data.
- Participant must have normal vision or corrected to normal vision.
- Participant must agree to sign a consent form, ensuring that they understood the details of the experiment; the form is provided in Appendix 2C.

13.5.3 Exclusion Criteria

- Fail to provide written consent (Appendix 2C).
- Fail to meet the requirements mentioned in inclusion criteria.

13.5.4 Sample Size Calculation

The minimum sample size was calculated using the statistical methods implemented in the PS (Power and Sample Size) software package and the computed sample size to achieve significant results in this study was 22 participants. The details of sample size calculation are briefly explained in Appendix 13A.

13.5.5 Experiment Design

Data collection was performed in a temperature-controlled environment (20–25°C) and a simulator-based driving environment was developed for the data acquisition. This study was conducted in collaboration with the MIROS and the driving simulator was provided by MIROS for the data acquisition. The data acquisition setup is shown in Fig. 13.2. The study protocol is presented in Fig. 13.3. The total time for the data collection of each participant was 3–4 hours, including signing of consent form, measuring blood pressure (BP), questionnaire completion, calibration of physiological data acquisition device, head measurement, and driving tasks. The whole experiment was performed on the same day for each participant.

The experiment consisted of five sessions: (1) preexperiment session, (2) familiarization drive (FD) session, (3) training drive (TD) session, (4) monotonous drive (MD) session, and (5) postexperiment session. In

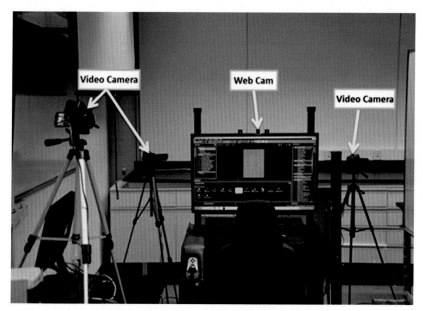

Figure 13.2 Experimental setup.

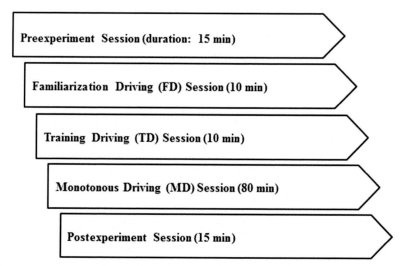

Preexperiment Session (duration: 15 min)

Familiarization Driving (FD) Session (10 min)

Training Driving (TD) Session (10 min)

Monotonous Driving (MD) Session (80 min)

Postexperiment Session (15 min)

Figure 13.3 Experimental protocol.

the preexperiment session, the participant's BP was measured. Additionally, each participant had given consent for the study to be performed and the participants were asked to complete a questionnaire related to drowsiness and mental states (see Appendix-13B). The next session was FD, in which participants drove the simulator-based car for 5–10 minutes. In this session, the participant was not wearing the physiological data acquisition device and the main aim was for the participant to familiarize themselves with the simulator, i.e., the road scenario, the force required to press the brake and the accelerator, and how to control the steering wheel. This session was followed by the TD session, in which the participant was wearing the data acquisition device and was allowed to drive for 10 minutes. This session mainly focused on getting the participant to feel comfortable with the EEG and ECG data acquisition device while driving.

Additionally, the participant was allowed to terminate the experiment if he/she experienced any issue such as headache, motion sickness, or physical sickness at any stage during data collection. The next session was the MD session, where the driver was asked to drive for 80 minutes. The driving scenario in this session was similar to driving on a highway in which there were no traffic signals and a very limited number of cars on the road. The vehicle speed was kept up to 80 km/hour to create a monotonous driving environment. Studies conducted in Refs. 16,17 showed that the time on task, nature of task, and vehicle speed are very important for getting drowsiness data. The last session was the postexperiment session, in which questions related to drowsiness, mental state, and the driving experiment were asked.

13.5.6 Precautions

Each participant was instructed to follow these experiment day precautions:
- Avoid usage of any kind of hair oil and gel on your head on the experiment day.
- Avoid any type of alcoholic drink 24 hours prior to the experiment.
- Avoid any type of caffeinated drinks (e.g., tea, coffee) 4 hours before starting the experiment.
- Avoid any kind of energy/carbonated drink 4 hours before starting the experiment.
- Avoid smoking 4 hours before starting the experiment.

13.6 DATA DESCRIPTION

EEG raw and clean data along with video recordings for one subject are provided with this book. The details of these files are provided in Table 13.2.

Table 13.2 EEG data description

S. No.	Directory name	EEG description
01	Eyes closed	This directory contains baseline eyes-closed EEG recordings in the file S1_EC.edf. There may be other supporting files created during data acquisition such as .info, .easy, .nedf. The readers should handle .edf file for analysis or data loading.
02	Baseline driving	This directory contains EEG file S1_TD.edf captured during the training drive for 10 min (baseline driving).
03	Monotonous driving	This directory contains EEG file S1_MD.edf, which was captured during monotonous drive for 80 min.

To access these files, please go to the directory BookData\Chap13\EEG for EEG data in the accompanied data files with this book. The EEG data files have an embedded ECG electrode (channel number 20). For the complete dataset of 22 subjects, please contact the authors at brainexpbook@gmail.com.

13.7 RELEVANT PAPERS

This section provides a list of some of the papers that have utilized the data acquired from the experiment described in this chapter. The following papers should be cited when using the experiment design or the data provided with this chapter.

1. Awais M, Badruddin N, Drieberg M. A non-invasive approach to detect drowsiness in a monotonous driving environment. In: *TENCON 2014–2014 IEEE Region 10 Conference*; 2014, pp. 1–4.
2. Awais M, Badruddin N, Drieberg M. Driver drowsiness detection using EEG power spectrum analysis. In: *Region 10 Symposium, 2014 IEEE*, 2014, pp. 244–247.

ACKNOWLEDGMENTS

This chapter provides the details of the experiment design available in the papers mentioned in Section 13.5.5 and in the MS thesis of Mr. M. Awais, which is available at Universiti Teknologi PETRONAS.

REFERENCES

1. Sahayadhas A, Sundaraj K, Murugappan M. Detecting driver drowsiness based on sensors: a review. *Sensors.* 2012;12(12):16937–16953.
2. Slater JD. A definition of drowsiness: one purpose for sleep? *Med Hypotheses.* 2008;71(5):641–644.
3. Traffic Safety Facts. 2010;854(March).
4. *State of the Road: Fatigue Fact Sheet.* Centre for Accident Research and Road Safety-Queensland (CARRS-Q), Australia 2011.
5. Annual Report of Malaysian Institute of Road Safety Research. 2007; http://www.miros.gov.my/.
6. Horne J, Reyner L. Vehicle accidents related to sleep: a review. *Occup Environ Med.* 1999;56(5):289–294.
7. Sagberg F. Road accidents caused by drivers falling asleep. *Accid Anal Prev.* 1999;31(6):639–649.
8. Mitler MM, Miller JC, Lipsitz JJ, Walsh JK, Wylie CD. The sleep of long-haul truck drivers. *N Engl J Med.* 1997;337(11):755–762.
9. Forsman PM, Vila BJ, Short RA, Mott CG, Van Dongen HPA. Efficient driver drowsiness detection at moderate levels of drowsiness. *Accid Anal Prev.* 2013;50:341–350.
10. Grace R, Steward S. Drowsy driver monitor and warning system. *Paper presented at: International driving symposium on human factors in driver assessment, training and vehicle design*; 2001.
11. Grace R, Byrne VE, Bierman DM, et al. A drowsy driver detection system for heavy vehicles. *Paper presented at: Digital Avionics Systems Conference, 1998. Proceedings., 17th DASC. The AIAA/IEEE/SAE*; 1998.
12. Moller HJ, Kayumov L, Bulmash EL, Nhan J, Shapiro CM. Simulator performance, microsleep episodes, and subjective sleepiness: normative data using convergent methodologies to assess driver drowsiness. *J Psychosom Res.* 2006;61(3):335–342.
13. Amin HU, Malik AS, Kamel N, Hussain M. A novel approach based on data redundancy for feature extraction of EEG signals. *Brain Topogr.* 2016;29(2):207–217.
14. Amin HU, Malik AS, Ahmad RF, et al. Feature extraction and classification for EEG signals using wavelet transform and machine learning techniques. *Australas Phys Eng Sci Med.* 2015;38(1):139–149.
15. Amin HU, Malik AS, Subhani AR, Badruddin N, Chooi W-T. Dynamics of scalp potential and autonomic nerve activity during intelligence test. In: Lee M, Hirose A, Hou Z-G, Kil R, editors. *Neural Information Processing,* Vol 8226. Heidelberg: Springer Berlin; 2013:9–16.
16. Thiffault P, Bergeron J. Monotony of road environment and driver fatigue: a simulator study. *Accid Anal Prev.* 2003;35(3):381–391.
17. Sahayadhas A, Sundaraj K, Murugappan M. Drowsiness detection during different times of day using multiple features. *Australas Phys Eng Sci Med.* 2013;36(2):243–250.

CHAPTER 14

Working Memory and Attention

Contents

14.1 INTRODUCTION

Memory is the mental ability to retain and recall past experience based on the cognitive processes of learning, retention, recall, and recognition. The process of forming new memories consists of three stages: encoding of new sensory information, retaining the encoded information over time, and recollection of stored memories. The process of encoding starts at birth and occurs continuously. Our senses pick up information to be memorized from our surroundings and send this information to short-term storage for manipulation; this is working memory (WM).[1] Important information that takes attention resources during manipulation goes into our long-term memory. There are several factors that can help to transfer information into long-term memory (see Ref. 2). The fundamentals of memory types, memory processes, and memory experimental paradigms can be seen in this review.[3]

The concept of WM was first proposed by Baddeley in 1974[4] with a model consisting of three main parts: the central executive, phonological loop, and visuospatial sketchpad. The WM manipulates and holds a limited amount of information for a limited time.[5] Some researchers believe that short-term storage and WM are the same, while others believe that

Designing EEG Experiments for Studying the Brain.
DOI: http://dx.doi.org/10.1016/B978-0-12-811140-6.00014-X
© 2017 Elsevier Inc.
All rights reserved.

short-term storage is essentially a part of WM, since it does not have the capabilities of manipulating the encoded information and it only holds the information for a limited time (<1 minutes).

But what is so important about WM? WM is the very first brain construct that processes the sensory information that comes through our senses into our brain and is sent to the frontal lobe for manipulation.[6] In the information processing in WM, much information is discarded and only required information is encoded to long-term storage. The performance of WM is crucial in all cognitive processes, especially in the learning process. Besides the significance and key role of WM in cognitive processes, it has some limitations, which are documented as follows:

1. The number of items that it can hold
2. The amount of time that these items can be held in WM

However, psychological studies revealed that not only are the number of items and the time period determining factors in measuring WM performance, but also attention can significantly influence its performance.[7,8] The definition of attention in its general form is *to selectively focus on a specific aspect of information while ignoring the other aspects.* To what extent this can be done is a significantly determining factor in WM performance. This is because regardless of the relevancy of the information, it will be held in WM; hence, attention plays a filtering role for the information that is being held in WM. If more irrelevant information can be inhibited, this will enhance the more relevant information and as a result WM ends up with a better performance since it is filled mostly with task-relevant information.

The mechanism that bridges between these two constructs is top-down modulation. Top-down modulation is when the processing command comes from higher processing units in brain to sensory parts, which is the case when we selectively (willingly) focus on something; in the case of interaction between attention and WM, we are selectively focusing on a specific task and observing the relevant information from it. That is why top-down modulation is the bridge between these two functionalities of the human brain. In contrast, a bottom–up mechanism is when something drives our attention toward itself.

14.2 IMPORTANCE OF STUDYING WORKING MEMORY ASSESSMENT

Attention and WM are two cognitive processes that have utmost importance in our daily life. In our surroundings, there is plenty of information coming through our senses into the brain. Not all sensory information is of interest to us. The brain perceives only that sensory information that is focused on or attended by the individual. Hence, attention is the process that helps one filter incoming sensory information, and the selected information is thus allowed into the WM manipulation.

WM is a process that uses existing information, manipulates it, and passes it to long-term memory if desired. However, there are individual differences in attention and WM capabilities.[9–11] Some studies reported the relationship of WM with general cognitive ability of fluid intelligence, i.e., WM may improve intelligence ability,[12] but there are also studies that reported that WM does not improve intelligence ability.[13] WM training has been reported to improve attention-deficit/hyperactivity disorder (ADHD) and other cognitive disorders.[14]

Besides the existing literature about the relationship of attention and WM for healthy individuals, it needs to be investigated further with the use of neuroimaging techniques such as EEG. The EEG experiments for WM and attention allow one to record time-locked EEG data and determine the neuronal changes during the experimental tasks. In the light of existing literature, the prefrontal and frontal regions are the hub of WM and attention-related activities. The connections of these locations with other brain regions in different individuals with different capabilities of these cognitive processes will be interesting to further explore.

14.3 PROBLEM STATEMENT

WM has been studied by researchers of psychology, neuroscience, and related disciplines using various brain imaging techniques such as electroencephalography (EEG) and functional magnetic resonance imaging (fMRI).[15,16] However, the significant role of attention in WM is still of considerable interest for researchers, especially the underlying neuronal mechanism of attention resources in information manipulation in WM.

In this experiment, we aimed to provide supporting evidence regarding the interaction between attention and WM and the neural activities that underlie the interaction between these two constructs.

Based on the problem statement mentioned previously, the objective of this study was to analyze the influence of attention in neural activities of the brain while performing a WM task. This can be examined in two different stages, i.e., encoding and maintenance. Hence, the objectives, in a clearer way, can be expressed as follows:

1. Analyze the influence of attention during the encoding stage on WM load (in the maintenance stage).

2. Analyze the behavior of WM in the maintenance stage while distraction and interruption is introduced through contralateral delay activity (CDA) during feature delayed response task.

14.4 SOFTWARE AND HARDWARE

See Table 14.1.

Table 14.1 Equipment and software

S. No.	Equipment/software	Description
01	BrainMaster amplifier	This amplifier supports 24 channels qEEG with the high-quality data required in research studies. It has 24-bit analog-to-digital converters. The 24 channels of EEG recording include 22 channels connected to a standard electrode cap, plus 2 channels of differential inputs with separate references, useful for monitoring any of a wide range of EEG or related potentials.
02	BrainMaster Discovery 24E	BrainMaster Discovery is acquisition software that supports the amplifier and can interface with the stimulus presentation software (E-Prime). The participant details can be entered in Discovery along with the experiment session, time, and date.
03	EEG caps (small, medium, large)	Electro-Caps are an EEG electrode application technique. They are made of an elastic spandex-type fabric with recessed, pure tin electrodes attached to the fabric. The electrodes on the standard caps are positioned to the international 10–20 method of electrode placement. The available sizes of Electro-Caps are 50–54 cm, 52–56 cm, 54–58 cm, 56–60 cm, and 58–62 cm.
04	Impedance meter	This includes a switch and associated circuitry to select up to 22 separate electrode leads. This allows the 1089ES to check applied electrode contact impedance of multiple electrode configurations such as the EEG 10–20 cap.
05	E-Prime 2.0	E-Prime software is used to construct the design of the experimental task. It provides feedback and time-lock events synchronized with the BrainMaster Discovery software to keep track of time events according to the stimulus presentation in the experiment.

14.5 EXPERIMENTAL DESIGN AND PROTOCOL

This section discusses the experimental design including the participant details, inclusion and exclusion criteria, sample size computation, design of memory task, and experiment procedure.

14.5.1 Target Population

In this study, the undergraduate students on the university campus were the target population. All the students on the university campus were the entire set of units for which the findings of the research had been generalized. Equal opportunity was given to all students who met the inclusion criteria to become a participant.

14.5.2 Sample Size Calculation

In terms of the first objective, the outcome of the study was to analyze WM performance with respect to filtering efficiency of the WM. This was achieved by looking at the changes in CDA amplitude with respect to the amount of distraction that was present in the stimuli, and at the same time we measured the WM performance by keeping track of the number of times the participant responded correctly.

Based on the literature, the amplitudes of CDA for stimuli with and without distraction are different. The result of the amplitude in two different situations is:

$$\left. \begin{array}{l} \text{Without distraction:} \quad 1.02 +/- 0.2865\,\mu V \\ \text{With distraction:} \quad\;\; 1.4344 +/- 0.4358\,\mu V \end{array} \right\} \boldsymbol{\delta = 0.4144,\ \sigma = 0.4358}$$

In terms of the second objective, the outcome of the research was to explore the behavior of CDA when distraction or interruption was presented while the encoded items were being maintained in WM. At the same time, the behavior of CDA could be correlated with the performance of WM, which was pretty close in these two cases. Hence, in this case, we used these percentages of WM performance as the basis to calculate a sample size that could be reliable to compare the performance of WM in these two different situations and be consistent to analyze the neural behavior of the brain as well. Hence we had:

1. No Interruption, No Distraction: 94.2% +/- 3%

2. With Distraction only: 91.6% +/- 2%

3. With Interruption only: 90.3% +/- 3%

Between 2 and 1: $\delta = 2.6$, $\sigma = 3$

Between 3 and 1: $\delta = 3.9$, $\sigma = 3$

The results were always compared with the reference, which was the no-interruption and no distraction condition. Having said that, the following formula[17] was used to compute the sample size for this experiment:

$$ n = \frac{2(Z_\alpha + Z_{1-\beta})^2 \sigma^2}{\delta^2} $$

In both cases, the significance level was 0.05, and power was 0.9. Since our test was one-tailed, the normal deviation (Z_α) for 0.05 significance level (Alpha) was 1.64, and normal deviation $Z_{(1-\beta)}$ for statistical power was 1.28. Putting this information and the previous information in the formula, the resulting sample size for each experiment was:

$$ \text{Objective 1: } n = \frac{2(1.64 + 1.28)^2 \times 0.4358^2}{0.4144^2} = 19 $$

$$ \text{Objective 2: } n = \frac{2(1.64 + 1.28)^2 \times 3^2}{2.6^2} = 23 $$

14.5.3 Experiment Design

In this experiment, a feature delayed response task was used. The description of the tasks is given in the following paragraphs.

14.5.3.1 Design of Task 1

In the first task (illustrated in Fig. 14.1), for the first objective, the participant must remember the position of the red cubes relative to each other. The only cubes to be remembered were the red color cubes. The color/number of distracting cubes might change. The cubes could be positioned in 18 different places in each visual field (VF). We limited the number of

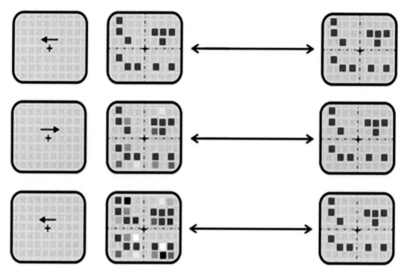

Figure 14.1 Design of experimental task 1.

red cubes to six, since it is believed that WM can hold items in the range of 7 ± 2,[1] depending on the content.

The number of red cubes was not altered throughout the experiment; only their position was changed. The attention of the participant was altered by adding different color cubes. As mentioned, each side can accommodate 18 cubes, since 6 spaces were filled with red cubes, there were 12 empty places left that could contain the distracting cubes with different colors. The colors of the distracting cubes varied between 7 colors (black, blue, lime, aqua, magenta, yellow, and white). The steps of the experiment can thus be described as follows:

Stimuli with no distraction. Six cubes in different positions were placed in each VF (12 in total image). The result of this experiment was used as the baseline/reference to compare the changes when distraction was introduced.

Stimuli with low distraction—4 (<6). In this step, the distracting cubes were added to the stimuli. The reason for choosing 4 was because we wanted to examine the brain activity when there were distracting cubes, but the number of distracting cubes was less than the red cubes. In other words, the intensity of distraction was low.

Stimuli with high distraction—8 (>6). In this step, we introduced more distraction as compared to the previous step, i.e., the number of nonred cubes was greater than the number of red cubes.

Please note that the number of red cubes was the same throughout the experiment. Only their position (relative to each other) was changed.

The participants were supposed to remember the position of the red cubes relative to each other as a whole pattern. In the testing array, the distractions would not appear, the reason being that the participants were asked to remember the position of red cubes and that is what they were going to be tested for. The point of introducing distraction was to alter the attention while encoding new information, and not to alter attention during retrieval.

The timing information of a single trial of task 1 is explained in Fig. 14.2. There were a total of 50 trials in task 1. Each trial started with a cue, presented for 200 ms, informing the participants to focus on a visual hemifield, either left or right. After the cue, the stimulus was presented for 300 ms (memory array) followed by a delayed period of duration of 1000 ms. Finally, the test array was displayed and the participants were required to respond by pressing a button if the test array matched with the memory array. There was a 2000-ms intertrial interval (ITI) between two consecutive trials.

In the second task (illustrated in Fig. 14.3), which was to achieve the second objective, there was no distraction or alteration of attention in the encoding stage; rather, we altered the attention during the maintenance stage through a combination of distraction and interruption (secondary task). Pictures were presented to participants containing red cubes; in case of distraction they must ignore, and in case of interruption they must perform a secondary task (explained below). In this task, as well as task 1, we had three (3) different levels. With respect to this explanation, the tasks were:

No distraction, no-interruption. In this case there was no distraction throughout the experiment; the result of this was used as a baseline/ reference to enable comparison with and analysis of the results of the other situations.

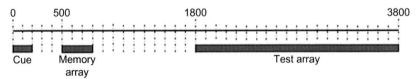

Figure 14.2 Explanation of timeline of task 1. Total time for one trial = 3800 ms Intertrial interval (ITI) = 2000 ms, Total time for one level (50 trials) = 3800 × 50 + 2000 × 49 = almost 5 min, Total time for task 1 = 5 × 3= 15 min (exclusive of breaks between levels).

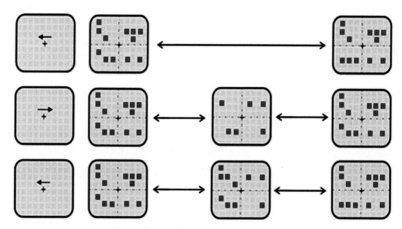

Figure 14.3 Design of experimental task 2.

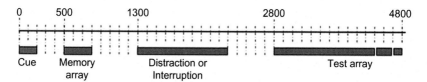

Figure 14.4 Explanation of timeline of task 2. Total time for one trial = 4800 ms Intertrial interval (ITI) = 2000 ms, Total time for one level (50 trials) = 4800 × 50 + 2000 × 49 = almost 6 min, Total time for task 2 = 6 × 3 = 18 min (exclusive of breaks between levels).

With distraction only. In this case, the stimulus containing cubes (same color with the cubes presented earlier in encoding stage) was presented to participants, and they were supposed to ignore it.

With interruption only. In this case, the stimulus containing cubes (same color) was presented to participants, and they were asked to distinguish whether the number of cubes (in the VF cued at the beginning of experiment) was more or less than 6. We chose 6 because that was the number of cubes presented in the encoding stage and it is a critical number in this case (at least more critical than other numbers).

The timing information of a single trial of task 2 is explained in Fig. 14.4. There were also a total of 50 trials in task 2. Each trial started with a cue, presented for 200 ms, informing the participants to focus on a visual hemifield, either left or right. After the cue, the stimulus was presented for 300 ms (memory array) followed by a delayed period of duration of 1000 ms. In this task, the delayed period was divided into two and in the middle a distraction or interruption image was displayed for 1000 ms. Finally, the test array was displayed and the participants were required to respond by pressing a button if the test array matched with the memory array. There was a 2000-ms ITI between two consecutive trials.

14.5.4 Experiment Procedure

All the participants were informed of the schedule of the data collection and as per their ease, experiments were arranged individually. Each participant was seated in a partially sound–attenuated experiment room and briefed about the experimental task before performing the actual experiment. The EEG cap was set and the participant was asked to perform the actual experimental task. The cap setting required 10–15 minutes.

14.6 DATA DESCRIPTION

EEG raw and clean data for one subject are provided with this book. The details of these files are provided in Table 14.2. To access the raw data files, please go to the directory BookData\Chapter14\EEGData\raw in the data files accompanying this book. For the complete dataset of 23 subjects, please contact the authors at brainexpbook@gmail.com. The experimental design files of E-Prime for both the WM tasks are provided in the directory BookData\Chap14\Design. These E-Prime files can only be opened when E-Prime is installed and the design can be understood with the help of information provided in Figs. 14.2 and 14.3.

14.6.1 EEG Description

See Table 14.2.

Table 14.2 Details of EEG data

S. No.	File name	EEG description
01	T1P1.edf	This file contains EEG data recorded during task 1. The number of trials and the duration of the task are mentioned in the design of task 1; see Fig. 14.2. The format of the file is .edf, which can be opened using MATLAB, EEGLAB, Neuroguide, and BESA software.
02	T2P1.edf	This file contains EEG data recorded during task 2. The number of trials and the duration of the task are mentioned in the design of task 2; see Fig. 14.3.

14.7 RELEVANT PAPERS

This section provides a list of some of the papers that have utilized the data acquired from the experiment described in this chapter. The following paper should be cited when using the experiment design or the data provided with this chapter.

1. Bashiri M, Mumtaz W, Malik AS, Waqar K. EEG-based brain connectivity analysis of working memory and attention. *Paper presented at: 2015 IEEE Student Symposium in Biomedical Engineering & Sciences (ISSBES)*; 2015.

ACKNOWLEDGMENTS

This chapter provides the details of the experiment design available in the papers mentioned in Section 14.6 and in the FYP report of Mohammad Bashiri, which is available at Universiti Teknologi PETRONAS.

REFERENCES

1. Baddeley A. Working memory: looking back and looking forward. *Nat Rev Neurosci.* 2003;4(10):829–839.
2. Amin HU, Malik AS. Memory retention and recall process. In: Kamel N, Malik AS, eds. *EEG/ERP Analysis: Methods and Applications*. London: CRC Press; 2014:219–237.
3. Amin H, Malik AS. Human memory retention and recall processes: a review of EEG and fMRI studies. *Neurosciences.* 2013;18(4):330–344.
4. Baddeley AD, Hitch G. Working memory. *Psychol Learn Motiv.* 1974;8:47–89.
5. Amin HU, Malik AS, Badruddin N, Chooi W-T. Brain activation during cognitive tasks: An overview of EEG and fMRI studies. *Paper presented at: Biomedical Engineering and Sciences (IECBES), 2012 IEEE EMBS Conference*; Malaysia; 2012.
6. Ahmad RF, Malik AS, Kamel N, Reza F, Abdullah JM. Simultaneous EEG-fMRI for working memory of the human brain. *Australas Phys Eng Sci Med.* 2016:1–16.
7. Engle RW. Working memory capacity as executive attention. *Curr Direct Psychol Sci.* 2002;11(1):19–23.
8. Awh E, Vogel E, Oh S-H. Interactions between attention and working memory. *Neuroscience.* 2006;139(1):201–208.
9. Engle RW, Kane MJ, Tuholski SW. Individual differences in working memory capacity and what they tell us about controlled attention, general fluid intelligence, and functions of the prefrontal cortex; 1999.
10. Vogel EK, Machizawa MG. Neural activity predicts individual differences in visual working memory capacity. *Nature.* 2004;428(6984):748–751.
11. Barrett LF, Tugade MM, Engle RW. Individual differences in working memory capacity and dual-process theories of the mind. *Psychol Bull.* 2004;130(4):553.
12. Jaeggi SM, Buschkuehl M, Jonides J, Perrig WJ. Improving fluid intelligence with training on working memory. *Proc Natl Acad Sci.* 2008;105(19):6829–6833.
13. Chooi W-T, Thompson LA. Working memory training does not improve intelligence in healthy young adults. *Intelligence.* 2012;40(6):531–542.
14. Melby-Lervåg M, Hulme C. Is working memory training effective? A meta-analytic review. *Dev Psychol.* 2013;49(2):270.

15. Cao H, Plichta MM, Schäfer A, et al. Test–retest reliability of fMRI-based graph theoretical properties during working memory, emotion processing, and resting state. *Neuroimage*. 2014;84(0):888–900.
16. Amin H, Malik A, Badruddin N, Chooi W-T. Brain behavior in learning and memory recall process: a high-resolution EEG analysis. In: Goh J, editor. *The 15th International Conference on Biomedical Engineering*, Vol 43. New York: Springer International Publishing; 2014:683–686.
17. Kadam P, Bhalerao S. Sample size calculation. *Int J Ayurveda Res*. 2010;1(1):55.

Appendices

APPENDIX 2A SUBJECT RECRUITMENT PRO FORMA SHEET

<u>**IMPORTANT NOTE:**</u> Filling this form does not mean that you are selected. You will be contacted in case you are shortlisted as a volunteer.

Participant Personal Information

Subject ID:

Contact Number: **E-mail:**

Gender: ☐ Male ☐ Female   **Race:**

Date of Birth: ___ (DD)/ ___ (MM)/ ___ (YY)   **Age:**

Questionnaire

1. Are you taking any daily medications?

   ☐ Yes   ☐ No

2. Do you have any current health problems of any sort (e.g.: diabetes, cancer, bed wetting, Etc.)?

   ☐ Yes   ☐ No

3. Have you ever experienced any head injury or brain disorder (e.g. epilepsy, seizures, migraine or any other)?

   ☐ Yes   ☐ No

4. Have you ever experienced any cardiac disorder (e.g heart attack, angina pain?)

   ☐ Yes   ☐ No

5. Do you have skin allergy?

   ☐ Yes   ☐ No

6. Do you smoke?

   ☐ Yes   ☐ No

7. How many hours do you usually sleep? Please tick ONE box only.

   ☐ less than 6 hours   ☐ 6 to 8 hours   ☐ more than 10 hours

8. How many hours per day (approximately) do you spend in front of a computer? Please tick ONE box only.

☐ less than 3 hours   ☐ 3 to 6 hours   ☐ 7to 10 hours   ☐ more than 10 hours

9. How many times per week do you see a movie?

10. How many times have you watched times 3D movies before?

11. Do you play video games? (Not at all,   not active player,   active player,   very active player)

12. Have you played Nintendo DS before?

      If yes, then please name the games that you have played.

13. Have you played Nintendo **3DS** before?

      If yes, then please name the games that you have played.

14. Have you played Sony Play-station before?

If yes, then please name the games that you have played.

15. Have you played 3D game using Sony Play-station 3?

If yes, then please name the games that you have played.

To Be Filled By The Authority

☐   Eligible to participate
☐   Not eligible to participate

APPENDIX 2B FEEDBACK QUESTIONNAIRE

1. Do you feel relaxed when answering task in the level?

   None   Slight   Moderate   Severe

2. Do you have enough time answering the arithmetic task? Rate it out of 10.

   1   2   3   4   5   6   7   8   9   10

3. Do you think before answering the task?

   None   Slight   Moderate   Severe

4. Do you answer the task randomly without knowing the right answer?

   None   Slight   Moderate   Severe

APPENDIX 2C SUBJECT INFORMATION AND CONSENT FORM

Subject Information and Consent Form
(Signature Page)

Research Title: _____

Researcher's Name: _____

To become a part this study, you or your legal representative must sign this page. By signing this page, I am confirming the following:

- I have read all of the information in this Subject Information and Consent Form **including any information regarding the risk in this study** and I have had time to think about it.
- All of my questions have been answered to my satisfaction.
- I voluntarily agree to be part of this research study, to follow the study procedures, and to provide necessary information to the doctor, nurses, or other staff members, as requested.
- I may freely choose to stop being a part of this study at anytime.
- I have received a copy of this Subject Information and Consent Form to keep for myself.

_____   _____
Subject Name (Print or type)   **Subject   Initials**   and
Number

_____   _____
Subject I.C No. (New)   **Subject   I.C** No.
(Old)

_____   _____
Signature of Subject or Legal Representative   **Date** (dd/MM/yy)
                                                    (Add time if applicable)
Ahmad Ruaf Subhani

_____
Name of Individual
Conducting Consent Discussion (Print or Type)

_____   _____
Signature of Individual   **Date** (dd/MM/yy)
Conducting Consent Discussion

_____   _____
Name & Signature of Witness   **Date** (dd/MM/yy)

<u>Note:</u>   i) All subject/subjects who are involved in this study will not be covered by insurance.

Subject's Material Publication Consent Form
Signature Page

Research Title: _____

Researcher's Name: _____

To become a part this study, you or your legal representative must sign this page.

By signing this page, I am confirming the following:

- I understood that my name will not appear on the materials published and there have been efforts to make sure that the privacy of my name is kept confidential although the confidentiality is not completely guaranteed due to unexpected circumstances.
- I have read the materials or general description of what the material contains and reviewed all photographs and figures in which I am included that could be published.
- I have been offered the opportunity to read the manuscript and to see all materials in which I am included, but have waived my right to do so.
- All the published materials will be shared among the medical practitioners, scientists and journalist worldwide.
- The materials will also be used in local publications, book publications and accessed by many local and international doctors worldwide.
- I hereby agree and allow the materials to be used in other publications required by other publishers with these conditions:
- The materials will not be used as advertisement purposes nor as packaging materials.
- The materials will not be used out of context – i.e.: Sample pictures will not be used in an article which is unrelated subject to the picture.

_____   _____

Subject Name (Print or type)   **Subject Initials** or **Number**

_____ _____   _____

Subject I.C No.   Subject's Signature   **Date** (dd/MM/yy)

_____   _____

Name and Signature of Individual   **Date** (dd/MM/yy)
Conducting Consent Discussion

<u>Note:</u> i) All subject/subjects who are involved in this study will not be covered by insurance.

APPENDIX 2D PERCEIVED STRESS SCALE (PSS) QUESTIONNAIRE

The questions in this scale ask you about your feelings and thoughts during the last month. In each case, you will be asked to indicate by circling how often you felt or thought a certain way.

Please provide fair information. Your information will be kept confidential.

Subject ID:					Date:	
Age:	Gender:		M/F			

0 = Never	1 = Almost Never	2 = Sometimes	3 = Fairly Often	4 = Very Often

		0	1	2	3	4
1	In the last month, how often have you been upset because of something that happened unexpectedly?					
2	In the last month, how often have you felt that you were unable to control the important things in your life?					
3	In the last month, how often have you felt nervous and stressed?					
4	In the last month, how often have you felt confident about your ability to handle your personal problems?					
5	In the last month, how often have you felt that things were going your way?					
6	In the last month, how often have you found that you could not cope with all the things that you had to do?					
7	In the last month, how often have you been able to control irritations in your life?					
8	In the last month, how often have you felt that you were on top of things?					
9	In the last month, how often have you been angered because of things that were outside of your control?					
10	In the last month, how often have you felt difficulties were piling up so high that you could not overcome them?					

Computing PSS Grade

The qualitative scale is labeled with numeric score from 0 (never) to 4 (very often). The scores for all questions accumulatively define a score that lies in one of four quartiles based on the severity of stress. These quartiles are 0–10, 11–14, 15–18, and 19–33,[7] where the first quartile represents no stress and the last quartile represents severe stress.

APPENDIX 3A HOSPITAL ANXIETY AND DEPRESSION SCALE (HADS)

Tick the box beside the reply that is closest to how you have been feeling in the past week.
Don't take too long thinking over your replies: your immediate reply is best.

D	A		D	A	
		I feel tense or "wound up":			**I feel as if I am slowed down:**
	3	Most of the time	3		Nearly all the time
	2	A lot of the time	2		Very often
	1	From time to time, occasionally	1		Sometimes
	0	Not at all	0		Not at all
		I still enjoy the things I used to enjoy:			**I get a sort of frightened feeling like "butterflies" in the stomach:**
0		Definitely as much		0	Not at all
1		Not quite so much		1	Occasionally
2		Only a little		2	Quite often
3		Hardly at all		3	Very often
		I get a sort of frightened feeling as if something awful is about to happen:			**I have lost interest in my appearance:**
	3	Very definitely and quite badly	3		Definitely
	2	Yes, but not too badly	2		I don't take as much care as I should
	1	A little, but it doesn't worry me	1		I may not take quite as much care
	0	Not at all	0		I take just as much care as ever
		I can laugh and see the funny side of things:			**I feel restless as I have to be on the move:**
0		As much as I always could		3	Very much indeed
1		Not quite so much now		2	Quite a lot
2		Definitely not so much now		1	Not very much
3		Not at all		0	Not at all
		Worrying thoughts go through my mind:			**I look forward with enjoyment to things:**
3		A great deal of the time		3	As much as I ever did
2		A lot of the time		2	Rather less than I used to
1		From time to time, but not too often		1	Definitely less than I used to
0		Only occasionally		0	Hardly at all
		I feel cheerful:			**I get sudden feelings of panic:**
3		Not at all		3	Very often indeed
2		Not often		2	Quite often
1		Sometimes		1	Not very often
0		Most of the time		0	Not at all
		I can sit at ease and feel relaxed:			**I can enjoy a good book or radio or TV program:**
	0	Definitely	0		Often
	1	Usually	1		Sometimes
	2	Not often	2		Not often
	3	Not at all	3		Very seldom

Please check that you have answered all the questions
Scoring: To compute the grade, simply accumulate all the scores entered by the participants in the range (0–3) and then compare with the following scale.
0–7 = Normal,
8–10 = Borderline abnormal (borderline case),
11–21 = Abnormal (case).

APPENDIX 3B BECK DEPRESSION INVENTORY-II (BDI-II)

This depression inventory can be self-scored. The scoring scale is at the end of the questionnaire.

1	0	I do not feel sad.
	1	I feel sad.
	2	I am sad all the time and I can't snap out of it.
	3	I am so sad and unhappy that I can't stand it.
2		
	0	I am not particularly discouraged about the future.
	1	I feel discouraged about the future.
	2	I feel I have nothing to look forward to.
	3	I feel the future is hopeless and that things cannot improve.
3		
	0	I do not feel like a failure.
	1	I feel I have failed more than the average person.
	2	As I look back on my life, all I can see is a lot of failures.
	3	I feel I am a complete failure as a person.
4		
	0	I get as much satisfaction out of things as I used to.
	1	I don't enjoy things the way I used to.
	2	I don't get real satisfaction out of anything anymore.
	3	I am dissatisfied or bored with everything.
5		
	0	I don't feel particularly guilty
	1	I feel guilty a good part of the time.
	2	I feel quite guilty most of the time.
	3	I feel guilty all of the time.
6		
	0	I don't feel I am being punished.
	1	I feel I may be punished.
	2	I expect to be punished.
	3	I feel I am being punished.
7		
	0	I don't feel disappointed in myself.
	1	I am disappointed in myself.
	2	I am disgusted with myself.
	3	I hate myself.
8		
	0	I don't feel I am any worse than anybody else.
	1	I am critical of myself for my weaknesses or mistakes.
	2	I blame myself all the time for my faults.
	3	I blame myself for everything bad that happens.

9		
	0	I don't have any thoughts of killing myself.
	1	I have thoughts of killing myself, but I would not carry them out.
	2	I would like to kill myself.
	3	I would kill myself if I had the chance.
10		
	0	I don't cry any more than usual.
	1	I cry more now than I used to.
	2	I cry all the time now.
	3	I used to be able to cry, but now I can't cry even though I want to.
11		
	0	I am no more irritated by things than I ever was.
	1	I am slightly more irritated now than usual.
	2	I am quite annoyed or irritated a good deal of the time.
	3	I feel irritated all the time.
12		
	0	I have not lost interest in other people.
	1	I am less interested in other people than I used to be.
	2	I have lost most of my interest in other people.
	3	I have lost all of my interest in other people.
13		
	0	I make decisions about as well as I ever could.
	1	I put off making decisions more than I used to.
	2	I have greater difficulty in making decisions more than I used to.
	3	I can't make decisions at all anymore.
14		
	0	I don't feel that I look any worse than I used to.
	1	I am worried that I am looking old or unattractive.
	2	I feel there are permanent changes in my appearance that make me look unattractive.
	3	I believe that I look ugly.
15		
	0	I can work about as well as before.
	1	It takes an extra effort to get started at doing something.
	2	I have to push myself very hard to do anything.
	3	I can't do any work at all.
16		
	0	I can sleep as well as usual.
	1	I don't sleep as well as I used to.
	2	I wake up 1–2 hours earlier than usual and find it hard to get back to sleep.
	3	I wake up several hours earlier than I used to and cannot get back to sleep.
17		
	0	I don't get more tired than usual.
	1	I get tired more easily than I used to.
	2	I get tired from doing almost anything.
	3	I am too tired to do anything.

18		
	0	My appetite is no worse than usual.
	1	My appetite is not as good as it used to be.
	2	My appetite is much worse now.
	3	I have no appetite at all anymore.
19		
	0	I haven't lost much weight, if any, lately.
	1	I have lost more than five pounds.
	2	I have lost more than ten pounds.
	3	I have lost more than fifteen pounds.
20		
	0	I am no more worried about my health than usual.
	1	I am worried about physical problems like aches, pains, upset stomach, or constipation.
	2	I am very worried about physical problems and it's hard to think of much else.
	3	I am so worried about my physical problems that I cannot think of anything else.
21		
	0	I have not noticed any recent change in my interest in sex.
	1	I am less interested in sex than I used to be.
	2	I have almost no interest in sex.
	3	I have lost interest in sex completely.

INTERPRETING THE BECK DEPRESSION INVENTORY

Now that you have completed the questionnaire, add up the score for each of the 21 questions by counting the number to the right of each question you marked. The highest possible total for the whole test would be 63. This would mean you circled number 3 on all 21 questions. Since the lowest possible score for each question is zero, the lowest possible score for the test would be zero. This would mean you circled zero on each question. You can evaluate your depression according to the table below.

Total score	Levels of depression
1–10	These ups and downs are considered normal
11–16	Mild mood disturbance
17–20	Borderline clinical depression
21–30	Moderate depression
31–40	Severe depression
Over 40	Extreme depression

APPENDIX 5A THE ALCOHOL USE DISORDERS IDENTIFICATION TEST

The Alcohol Use Disorders Identification Test (AUDIT) was developed by the World Health Organization for detecting people with harmful drinking status. It is also used for screening for alcoholics. The AUDIT for alcohol consumption (AUDIT-C), or the short version of AUDIT with only the first three questions, can be used as a screening test for problem drinking only. The details of AUDIT are illustrated in the table of questions below:

1	How often do you have a drink containing alcohol?	Never/Monthly or less/2–4 times a month/2–3 times a week/4 or more times a week
2	How many standard drinks containing alcohol do you have on typical day when drinking?	1 or 2/3 or 4/5 or 6/7 or 9/10 or more
3	How often do you have six or more drinks on one occasion?	Never/Less than monthly/ Monthly/Weekly/Daily or almost daily
4	During the past year, how often have you found that you were not able to stop drinking once you had started?	Never/Less than monthly/ Monthly/Weekly/Daily or almost daily
5	During the past year, how often have you failed to do what was normally expected of you because of drinking?	Never/Less than monthly/ Monthly/Weekly/Daily or almost daily
6	During the past year, how often have you needed a drink in the morning to get yourself going after a heavy drinking session?	Never/Less than monthly/ Monthly/Weekly/Daily or almost daily
7	During the past year, how often have you had the feeling of guilt or remorse after drinking?	Never/Less than monthly/ Monthly/Weekly/Daily or almost daily
8	During the past year, have you been unable to remember what happened the night before because you had been drinking?	Never/Less than monthly/ Monthly/Weekly/Daily or almost daily
9	Have you or someone else been injured as a result of your drinking?	No/Yes, but not in the past year/ Yes, during the past year
10	Has a relative or friend, doctor, or other health worker been concerned about your drinking or suggested you cut down?	No/Yes, but not in the past year/ Yes, during the past year

Each question will be scored from 0 to 4 depending on the answers. Then, to determine if the person has problem with their drinking status or not, all the scores will be summed up and interpreted using the scale as shown in the table below:

Score of	Means
0–7	Low risk of alcohol-related harm
8–10	High risk or experiencing alcohol-related harm (some people in this range will already be experiencing significant harm)
11–19	A person scoring in this range will already be experiencing significant alcohol-related harm
20+	A person scoring in this range may be alcohol dependent and is advised to see a health care professional about their drinking

APPENDIX 5B MINI INTERNATIONAL NEUROPSYCHIATRIC INTERVIEW (MINI)

J. ALCOHOL ABUSE AND DEPENDENCE

(➡ MEANS: GO TO DIAGNOSTIC BOXES, CIRCLE NO IN BOTH AND MOVE TO THE NEXT MODULE)

		➡	
J1	**In the past 12 months**, have you had 3 or more alcoholic drinks within a 3 hour period on 3 or more occasions?	NO	YES

J2   **In the past 12 months:**

a   Did you need to drink more in order to get the same effect that you got when you first started drinking?   NO   YES

b   When you cut down on drinking did your hands shake, did you sweat or feel agitated? Did you drink to avoid these symptoms or to avoid being hungover, for example, "the shakes", sweating or agitation?
IF YES TO EITHER, CODE YES.   NO   YES

c   During the times when you drank alcohol, did you end up drinking more than you planned when you started?   NO   YES

d   Have you tried to reduce or stop drinking alcohol but failed?   NO   YES

e   On the days that you drank, did you spend substantial time in obtaining alcohol, drinking, or in recovering from the effects of alcohol?   NO   YES

f   Did you spend less time working, enjoying hobbies, or being with others because of your drinking?   NO   YES

g   Have you continued to drink even though you knew that the drinking caused you health or mental problems?   NO   YES

ARE **3** OR MORE **J2** ANSWERS CODED **YES**?

* IF YES, SKIP J3 QUESTIONS, CIRCLE N/A IN THE ABUSE BOX AND MOVE TO THE NEXT DISORDER. DEPENDENCE PREEMPTS ABUSE.

NO	YES*
ALCOHOL DEPENDENCE CURRENT	

J3   **In the past 12 months:**

a   Have you been intoxicated, high, or hungover more than once when you had other responsibilities at school, at work, or at home? Did this cause any problems?
(CODE YES ONLY IF THIS CAUSED PROBLEMS.)   NO   YES

b   Were you intoxicated more than once in any situation where you were physically at risk, for example, driving a car, riding a motorbike, using machinery, boating, etc.?   NO   YES

c   Did you have legal problems more than once because of your drinking, for example, an arrest or disorderly conduct?   NO   YES

d   Did you continue to drink even though your drinking caused problems with your family or other people?   NO   YES

ARE **1** OR MORE **J3** ANSWERS CODED **YES**?

NO	N/A	YES
ALCOHOL ABUSE CURRENT		

APPENDIX 5C ALCOHOL WITHDRAWAL ASSESSMENT SCORING GUIDELINES (CIWA-Ar)

Alcohol Withdrawal Assessment Scoring Guidelines (CIWA - Ar)

Nausea/Vomiting - Rate on scale 0 - 7

0 - None
1 - Mild nausea with no vomiting
2
3
4 - Intermittent nausea
5
6
7 - Constant nausea and frequent dry heaves and vomiting

Tremors - have patient extend arms & spread fingers. Rate on scale 0 - 7.

0 - No tremor
1 - Not visible, but can be felt fingertip to fingertip
2
3
4 - Moderate, with patient's arms extended
5
6
7 - severe, even w/ arms not extended

Anxiety - Rate on scale 0 - 7

0 - no anxiety, patient at ease
1 - mildly anxious
2
3
4 - moderately anxious or guarded, so anxiety is inferred
5
6
7 - equivalent to acute panic states seen in severe delirium or acute schizophrenic reactions.

Agitation - Rate on scale 0 - 7

0 - normal activity
1 - somewhat normal activity
2
3
4 - moderately fidgety and restless
5
6
7 - paces back and forth, or constantly thrashes about

Paroxysmal Sweats - Rate on Scale 0 - 7.

0 - no sweats
1- barely perceptible sweating, palms moist
2
3
4 - beads of sweat obvious on forehead
5
6
7 - drenching sweats

Orientation and clouding of sensorium - Ask, "What day is this? Where are you? Who am I?" Rate scale 0 - 4

0 - Oriented
1 – cannot do serial additions or is uncertain about date

2 - disoriented to date by no more than 2 calendar days

3 - disoriented to date by more than 2 calendar days
4 - Disoriented to place and / or person

Tactile disturbances - Ask, "Have you experienced any itching, pins & needles sensation, burning or numbness, or a feeling of bugs crawling on or under your skin?"
0 - none
1 - very mild itching, pins & needles, burning, or numbness
2 - mild itching, pins & needles, burning, or numbness
3 - moderate itching, pins & needles, burning, or numbness
4 - moderate hallucinations
5 - severe hallucinations
6 - extremely severe hallucinations
7 - continuous hallucinations

Auditory Disturbances - Ask, "Are you more aware of sounds around you? Are they harsh? Do they startle you? Do you hear anything that disturbs you or that you know isn't there?"
0 - not present
1 - Very mild harshness or ability to startle
2 - mild harshness or ability to startle
3 - moderate harshness or ability to startle
4 - moderate hallucinations
5 - severe hallucinations
6 - extremely severe hallucinations
7 - continuous hallucinations

Visual disturbances - Ask, "Does the light appear to be too bright? Is its color different than normal? Does it hurt your eyes? Are you seeing anything that disturbs you or that you know isn't there?"
0 - not present
1 - very mild sensitivity
2 - mild sensitivity
3 - moderate sensitivity
4 - moderate hallucinations
5 - severe hallucinations
6 - extremely severe hallucinations
7 - continuous hallucinations

Headache - Ask, "Does your head feel different than usual? Does it feel like there is a band around your head?" Do not rate dizziness or lightheadedness.

0 - not present
1 - very mild
2 - mild
3 - moderate
4 - moderately severe
5 - severe
6 - very severe
7 - extremely severe

Procedure:

1. Assess and rate each of the 10 criteria of the CIWA scale. Each criterion is rated on a scale from 0 to 7, except for "Orientation and clouding of sensorium" which is rated on scale 0 to 4. Add up the scores for all ten criteria. This is the total CIWA-Ar score for the patient at that time. Prophylactic medication should be started for any patient with a total CIWA-Ar score of 8 or greater (ie. start on withdrawal medication). If started on scheduled medication, additional PRN medication should be given for a total CIWA-Ar score of 15 or greater.

2. Document vitals and CIWA-Ar assessment on the Withdrawal Assessment Sheet. Document administration of PRN medications on the assessment sheet as well.

3. The CIWA-Ar scale is the most sensitive tool for assessment of the patient experiencing alcohol withdrawal. Nursing assessment is vitally important. Early intervention for CIWA-Ar score of 8 or greater provides the best means to prevent the progression of withdrawal.

Assessment Protocol	**Date**												
a. Vitals, Assessment Now.	**Time**												
b. If initial score ≥ 8 repeat q1h x 8 hrs, then if stable q2h x 8 hrs, then if stable q4h.													
c. If initial score < 8, assess q4h x 72 hrs. If score < 8 for 72 hrs, d/c assessment.	**Pulse**												
If score ≥ 8 at any time, go to (b) above.	**RR**												
d. If indicated, (see indications below) administer prn medications as ordered and record on MAR and below.	**O2 sat**												
	BP												

Assess and rate each of the following (CIWA-Ar Scale):	Refer to reverse for detailed instructions in use of the CIWA-Ar scale.												
Nausea/vomiting (0 - 7) 0 - none; 1 - mild nausea ,no vomiting; 4 - intermittent nausea; 7 - constant nausea , frequent dry heaves & vomiting.													
Tremors (0 - 7) 0 - no tremor; 1 - not visible but can be felt; 4 - moderate w/ arms extended; 7 - severe, even w/ arms not extended.													
Anxiety (0 - 7) 0 - none, at ease; 1 - mildly anxious; 4 - moderately anxious or guarded; 7 - equivalent to acute panic state													
Agitation (0 - 7) 0 - normal activity; 1 - somewhat normal activity; 4 - moderately fidgety/restless; 7 - paces or constantly thrashes about													
Paroxysmal Sweats (0 - 7) 0 - no sweats; 1 - barely perceptible sweating, palms moist; 4 - beads of sweat obvious on forehead; 7 - drenching sweat													
Orientation (0 - 4) 0 - oriented; 1 - uncertain about date; 2 - disoriented to date by no more than 2 days; 3 - disoriented to date by > 2 days; 4 - disoriented to place and / or person													
Tactile Disturbances (0 - 7) 0 - none; 1 - very mild itch, P&N, ,numbness; 2-mild itch, P&N, burning, numbness; 3 - moderate itch, P&N, burning ,numbness; 4 - moderate hallucinations; 5 - severe hallucinations; 6 - extremely severe hallucinations; 7 - continuous hallucinations													
Auditory Disturbances (0 - 7) 0 - not present; 1 - very mild harshness/ ability to startle; 2 - mild harshness, ability to startle; 3 - moderate harshness, ability to startle; 4 - moderate hallucinations; 5 severe hallucinations; 6 - extremely severe hallucinations; 7 - continuous.hallucinations													
Visual Disturbances (0 - 7) 0 - not present; 1 - very mild sensitivity; 2 - mild sensitivity; 3 - moderate sensitivity; 4 - moderate hallucinations; 5 - severe hallucinations; 6 - extremely severe hallucinations; 7 - continuous hallucinations													
Headache (0 - 7) 0 - not present; 1 - very mild; 2 - mild; 3 - moderate; 4 - moderately severe; 5 - severe; 6 - very severe; 7 - extremely severe													
Total CIWA-Ar score:													
PRN Med: (circle one) Diazepam Lorazepam **Dose given (mg):** **Route:**													
Time of PRN medication administration:													
Assessment of response (CIWA-Ar score 30-60 minutes after medication administered)													
RN Initials													

Scale for Scoring:
Total Score =

    0 – 9: absent or minimal withdrawal
    10 – 19: mild to moderate withdrawal
    more than 20: severe withdrawal

Patient Identification (Addressograph)

Indications for PRN medication:
  a. Total CIWA-AR score 8 or higher if ordered PRN only (Symptom-triggered method).
  b. Total CIWA-Ar score 15 or higher if on Scheduled medication. (Scheduled + prn method)
  Consider transfer to ICU for any of the following: Total score above 35, q1h assess. x more than 8hrs required, more than 4 mg/hr lorazepam x 3hr **or** 20 mg/hr diazepam x 3hr required, or resp. distress.

Signature/ Title	Initials	Signature / Title	Initials

Alcohol Withdrawal Assessment Flowsheet (revised Nov 2003)

APPENDIX 6A DEMOGRAPHIC DATA

Demographic data for 40 subjects

Subject ID	Group[a]	Age[b]	Gender[c]	Handedness[d]	Experience in 3D[e]
A01	0	21	1	1	1
A02	0	22	1	1	1
A03	0	20	1	1	1
A04	0	21	1	2	1
A05	0	22	1	1	1
A06	0	19	1	1	1
A07	0	21	1	1	1
A08	0	22	2	1	1
A09	0	21	2	1	1
A10	0	20	1	1	1
A11	0	23	2	1	1
A12	0	21	2	1	1
A13	0	19	2	1	1
A14	0	22	1	1	1
A15	0	24	1	1	1
A16	0	22	1	2	1
A17	0	21	1	1	1
A18	0	20	1	1	1
A19	0	19	1	1	1
A20	0	23	1	1	1
P01	1	21	1	1	1
P02	1	21	1	1	1
P03	1	22	1	1	1
P04	1	21	1	1	1
P05	1	21	1	1	1
P06	1	20	1	1	1
P07	1	21	1	1	1
P08	1	25	1	2	1
P09	1	19	2	1	1
P10	1	22	2	1	1
P11	1	21	1	1	1
P12	1	21	1	1	1
P13	1	21	2	1	1
P14	1	22	1	1	1
P15	1	22	2	1	1
P16	1	23	2	1	1
P17	1	24	1	1	1
P18	1	24	1	1	1
P19	1	24	1	1	1
P20	1	24	1	1	1

[a]Group (0 = 3D Active first; 1 = 3D Passive first).
[b]Age in years.
[c]Gender (1 = Male; 2 = Female).
[d]Handedness (1 = Right; 2 = Left).
[e]Experience in 3D (1 = Yes; 2 = No).

Age descriptions of 40 subjects

Group	Number of subjects, N	Range[a]	Mean	SD[b]
3D Active first	20	19–24	21.15	1.3870
3D Passive first	20	19–25	21.95	1.5720
Total	40	19–25	21.55	1.5183

[a]Age range in years.
[b]SD = Standard Deviation

Cross-tabulation of experimental group, gender, and handedness of 40 subjects with column percentage in parentheses

Group	Gender		Handedness		Total
	Male	Female	Right	Left	
3D Active first	15 (50%)	5 (50%)	18 (48.6%)	2 (66.7%)	20 (50%)
3D Passive first	15 (50%)	5 (50%)	19 (51.4%)	1 (33.3%)	20 (50%)
Total	30	10	37	3[a]	40

[a]All left-handed subjects are male.

APPENDIX 6B SIMULATOR SICKNESS QUESTIONNAIRE (SSQ) AND FEEDBACK FORM

Post – Test: Simulator Sickness Questionnaire (SSQ)

Subject ID: _____   Experiment: 2D / 3D Active/ 3D Passive

Please CIRCLE ONLY ONE answer for each symptom to indicate your experience as of what you are feeling right now.

Example:

| 1 | General discomfort | None | Slight | Moderate | Severe |

No.	Symptom	Severity of the symptom			
1	General discomfort	None	Slight	Moderate	Severe
2	Fatigue	None	Slight	Moderate	Severe
3	Headache	None	Slight	Moderate	Severe
4	Eyestrain	None	Slight	Moderate	Severe
5	[a]Difficulty focusing	None	Slight	Moderate	Severe
6	Increased salivation	None	Slight	Moderate	Severe
7	Sweating	None	Slight	Moderate	Severe
8	Nausea	None	Slight	Moderate	Severe
9	Difficulty concentrating	None	Slight	Moderate	Severe
10	Fullness of head	None	Slight	Moderate	Severe
11	Blurred vision	None	Slight	Moderate	Severe
12	Dizziness with eyes open	None	Slight	Moderate	Severe
13	Dizziness with eyes closed	None	Slight	Moderate	Severe
14	[b]Vertigo	None	Slight	Moderate	Severe
15	[c]Stomach awareness	None	Slight	Moderate	Severe
16	Burping	None	Slight	Moderate	Severe

[a]Difficulty focusing on close objects (vision)
[b]Vertigo is a loss of orientation with respect to vertical upright
[c]Stomach awareness is temporary discomfort which is just short of nausea

*** END OF QUESTIONNAIRE ***

The procedure for computing column score in SSQ is provided as follows:

No.	Symptom	Nausea[a]	Oculomotor[b]	Disorientation[c]
1	General discomfort	1	1	0
2	Fatigue	0	1	0
3	Headache	0	1	0
4	Eyestrain	0	1	0
5	Difficulty focusing	0	1	1
6	Increased salivation	1	0	0
7	Sweating	1	0	0
8	Nausea	1	0	1
9	Difficulty concentrating	1	1	0
10	Fullness of head	0	0	1
11	Blurred vision	0	1	1
12	Dizziness with eyes open	0	0	1
13	Dizziness with eyes closed	0	0	1
14	Vertigo	0	0	1
15	Stomach awareness	1	0	0
16	Burping	1	0	0

Total SSQ score = $(A + B + C) \times 3.74$.
[a]Scale multiplication factor: Nausea: $A = score \times 9.54$.
[b]Oculomotor: $B = score \times 7.58$.
[c]Disorientation: $C = score \times 13.92$.

Post – Questionnaire/ Feedback

Subject ID: _____

Please CIRCLE ONLY ONE answer for each question to indicate your experience as of what you are feeling right now.

Example: 1. Did you feel energized because of 3D?

None   (Slightly)   Moderate   Severe

• •

1. Do you feel energized because of 3D?

None   Slightly   Moderate   Severe

2. Do you have a general feeling of discomfort/ exhaustion because of 3D?

None   Slightly   Moderate   Severe

3. Do you prefer watching movie in 3D than in 2D?

None   Slightly   Moderate   Severe

4. Would you want to watch 3D movie again?

None   Slightly   Moderate   Severe

5. Would you encourage 3D application in education and learning?

None   Slightly   Moderate   Severe

6. Do you prefer watching 3D movies with 3D Active or 3D Passive system? Please explain.

3D Active Shutter system   3D Passive Polarized system

because … ....

*** END OF QUESTIONNAIRE ***

APPENDIX 7A SCREENING QUESTIONNAIRE

SCREENING QUESTIONNAIRE

Participant's ID:_____Gender (M/F):_____Date of Birth:_____

Age:_____Qualification:_____Grade/GPA/%age:_____

Handedness (L/R):_____Contact No:_____Email:_____

S. No.	Questions	Response	
1	Are you currently taking any drugs that might affect your memory, hearing, vision, or motor skills (e.g., alcohol)?	Yes	No
2	Do you have any uncorrected vision impairment?	Yes	No
3	Do you have any uncorrected hearing impairments?	Yes	No
4	Have you have suffered any head injury?	Yes	No
5	Have you ever been diagnosed with an affective disorder (e.g., depression, bipolar depression)?	Yes	No
7	Are you currently suffering from any conditions like headaches, forgetfulness etc.?	Yes	No
8	Do you have any skin allergies or sensitivities?	Yes	No
9	Are you currently taking any medications?	Yes	No
10	Do you feel well rested from last night's sleep?	Yes	No

Excluded Criteria: *If any of the participant's responses falls in a shaded option, then the participant will be excluded from the study* (this line will be removed from the participant)

APPENDIX 7B FEEDBACK QUESTIONNAIRE

Feedback Questionnaire

Participant's ID:_____ Experiment Group:_____

Date: _____ Gender:_____

5	4	3	2	1
Strongly Agree	Agree	Unknown	Disagree	Strongly Disagree

Note: Please tick (√) one of the appropriate boxes for each questions.

S. No.	Questions	Responses				
		5	4	3	2	1
1.	Do you think that the contents are readable?					
2.	Do you think that the contents are easy to understand?					
3.	Did you feel any fatigue in your eyes during the experiment?					
4.	Do you think that the contents are meaningful?					
5.	Do you remember the items in the experiment easily?					

Comments:

_____

_____

_____

_____

_____

APPENDIX 9A QUESTIONNAIRE

<u>Questionnaire</u>

The purpose of this survey is to assess your level of familiarity with video games and your gaming habits. Please read each question carefully and answer as accurately as possible. Your response to each question represents a critical aspect of this research, so please try to answer each question as best you can. If you have any questions, please ask the experimenter.

Name:_____   E-mail:_____

Phone number:_____ Age:_____ Sex:_____   ID number:_____

Handedness:_____Right-handed   Left-Handed

Please circle one answer per question.

How many times in the past year have you done the following:

1. Played a PC-based video game?

Never   Seldom   Sometimes   Frequently   Often

2. Played a console video game system (e.g., Playstation 3, Game Cube, X-Box, etc...)?

Never   Seldom   Sometimes   Frequently   Often

3. Played a video game in an arcade?

Never   Seldom   Sometimes   Frequently   Often

4. Do you consider yourself to be an active video game player?

Yes   No

5. During an average week, how many hours will you spend playing video games?

<1 hour   1–3 hours   3–5 hours   5–7 hours   7–9 hours   >9 hours

6. How often did you play video games as a child?

Never   Seldom   Sometimes   Frequently   Often

7. Do you own a personal computer?

Yes   No

Specific Game Experience:

How frequently do you do the following:

1.   Play DOOM, Quake, Halo, Half-Life, or similar first-person shooters?

Never   Seldom   Sometimes   Frequently   Often

2.   Play Starcraft, Warcraft, Command and Conquer, Age of Empires, Civilization, Sim City, or similar strategy games?

Never   Seldom   Sometimes   Frequently   Often

3.   I consider myself:
     A.   A non–video game player
     B.   A novice video game player
     C.   An occasional video game player
     D.   A frequent video game player
     E.   An expert video game player

4.   Compared to five years ago:
     A.   I play video games more frequently now.
     B.   I play video games less frequently now.
     C.   There has been little change in the frequency of my video game playing.

Health-Related Issues:

1.   Have you ever experienced an electroencephalography (EEG) test before?
     Yes   No
2.   Are you taking any daily medications?
     Yes   No
3.   Do you have any current health problems?
     Yes   No
4.   Have you ever experienced any form of severe head injury or very high fever?
     Yes   No
5.   Do you have a skin allergy?
     Yes   No
6.   Do you have normal or corrected-to-normal vision?
     Yes   No

APPENDIX 10A EYE EXAMINATION FORM

A) DemographicData   Date:_____

1. IC NO :_____   Research ID _____

2. Age   : _____Years

3. Sex   : M / F

4. Race: Malay   ☐

        Chinese   ☐

        India   ☐

        Others   ☐

5. History of Motion Sickness: Yes/No

6. Past Medical History

    DM   ☐

    HPT   ☐

    IHD   ☐

    Asthma   ☐

	RIGHT	LEFT
Visual Acuity		
Refraction		

B) Eye Examination

RIGHT EYE		PUPIL	LEFT EYE	
	Cornea	ANTERIOR SEGMENT	Cornea	
	Anterior Chamber		Anterior Chamber	
FUNDUS			FUNDUS	
	Colour		Colour	
	CDR	OPTIC DISC	CDR	
		MACULA		
		PERIPHERY		

APPENDIX 10B MOTION SICKNESS SUSCEPTIBILITY QUESTIONNAIRE

Demographic data   **English form**

Date: _____

1	First name	
2	Last name	
3	Gender	
4	Email	
5	Age	
6	Phone no.	
7	Handedness	
8	Nationality	
9	Race	
10	Eyesight (Y/N) if "Y" state the power	
11	Daily medication (Y/N)	
12	Smoking (Y/N)	
13	Neurological disease (epilepsy, seizures, or migraine) (Y/N)	
14	Systemic problem (asthma, blood pressure, hypertension, or diabetes) (Y/N)	
15	Eye disease or surgery (Y/N)	
16	Ear problem or surgery (Y/N)	
17	Watched 3D within last 3 months (Y/N)	
18	Semester	

Motion Sickness Susceptibility Questionnaire Short Form (MSSQ—Short)
Please indicate in the appropriate sections your **childhood** experience only (before 12 years of age), and your **adult** experience over the last 10 years (approximately), for each of the following types of transport or entertainment.
For example, if you have never traveled in a car, then tick the **Never traveled** box under Cars. If you have felt sick sometimes while traveling in a car, then tick the **Sometimes felt sick** box under Cars.

Childhood	never travelled	Never felt sick	Rarely felt sick	sometimes felt sick	frequently felt sick
Cars					
Busses					
Trains					
Aircraft					
Small boats					
Ships e.g. channel ferries					
Swings in playgrounds					
Roundabouts in playgrounds					
Big dippers, Funfair rides					

Adult	never travelled	Never felt sick	Rarely felt sick	sometimes felt sick	frequently felt sick
Cars					
Busses					
Trains					
Aircraft					
Small boats					
Ships eg channel ferries					
Swings in playgrounds					
Roundabouts in playgrounds					
Big dippers, Funfair rides					

APPENDIX 11A QUESTIONNAIRE FORM

QUESTIONNARE FORM

Participant	Personal

Name:

Contact Number: **E-mail:**

Gender: Male ☐   Female ☐

Age:

Questionnaire

1. Have you ever experienced an EEG test before?

    Yes ☐   No ☐

2. Are you taking any daily medications?

    Yes ☐   No ☐

3. Do you have any current health problems of any sort (e.g.: diabetes, cancer, bed wetting, Etc.)?

    Yes ☐   No ☐

4. Have you ever experienced any form of severe head injury/ severfever?

    YES ☐   NO ☐

5. Do you have skin allergy?

    YES ☐   NO ☐

6. How many calls you normally have per day?

_____

7. What is the average duration per call?

_____

8. What are the effects that you usually have when using mobile phone?

_____

9. How long these effects usually last?

_____

10. Are you suffer from any permanent headache?

_____

11. If yes, how many times you suffer from it? (Per week or per month)

_____

APPENDIX 13A SAMPLE SIZE CALCULATION

Sample information: Single group of normal people.

Experiment conditions

One condition: monotonous driving with 80 km/h as a maximum speed limit

Test criteria:

1. Significance level $\alpha = 0.05$ for 95% significance (in this case we will be using a two-tailed test because the results could be bidirectional)
2. Power = 80% to reject null hypothesis.

The calculated number of participants to be included in the study is from 7 to 19. However, in practice we have to recruit more subjects to account for the possible dropouts. For sample size calculation, PS software is used with paired *t*-test[1] (Table A.1).

Table A.1 List of sample size studies

Reference	Calculated sample size with test criteria	Sample size
Lal et al.[2]	Lal et al. documented the differences of matched pairs as Gaussian distributed and reported the standard deviation (SD) as 0.86. To reject the null hypothesis, i.e., zero response difference with 80% statistical power in this study, the investigators require 14 pairs of subjects for a true difference in mean response of 0.7. In this experiment, the alpha value (type I error probability) is kept 0.05.	14
Lal et al.[2]	Lal et al. reported the normally distributed mean difference in response of matched pairs 3.07 value for standard deviation. The investigators computed the sample size, which is 16 pairs of participants, to prove the rejection of the null hypothesis (i.e., zero mean difference in response of matched pairs) if the reported true difference in mean response of matched pairs is 2.3. The investigators used 80% statistical power and 0.05 alpha values.	16

(Continued)

Table A.1 List of sample size studies (Continued)

Reference	Calculated sample size with test criteria	Sample size
Patel et al.[3]	Patel et al. reported the standard deviation 0.87 from their experimental results and normal distributed mean difference in the response of matched pairs. The investigators need to include 19 pairs of subjects to show the rejection of zero mean difference in response with 80% statistical power and 0.05 type I error probability, if the reported true mean difference in response is 0.6.	19
Cantero et al.[4]	Cantero et al. studied with standard deviation 0.04 and normal distributed mean difference in their investigation. The investigators of this study may require 7 pairs of participants to reject the null hypothesis with the same alpha value and statistical power as mentioned in the above three cases.	7

APPENDIX 13B   DROWSINESS QUESTIONNAIRE

Sleep and Monotonous Driving Condition   Subject No. : _____
Effect in Driving Simulator/Driver Drowsiness Detection using Physiological Signals

Part A: Personal Particular

Age: _____ years

Male ☐   Female ☐

Height: _____ m
Weight: _____ kg   BMI : _____

Blood pressure : _____ mm / _____ Hg

Occupation:
    Student   ☐
    Profesional and management   ☐
    Support   ☐
    Not working   ☐

In last 3 hours, how much do you:
    Smoke   _____ cigaratte/s
    Consume caffein   _____ cup/s
    Consume alcohol   _____ glass/es

Are you on medication?   Yes ☐   No ☐

Health history:
    Migrain   ☐
    Gastric   ☐
    Epilepsy   ☐
    High blood pressure   ☐

Driving experience: _____ years

No. of crashes involved as a driver in past 3
years: _____ crashes

No. of near crashes involved as a driver in past 3
years: _____ crashes

Crashes / near crashes caused by drowsiness:
    Crashes: _____ cases
    Near crashes: _____ cases

Part B: Current Sleepiness Level

Based on following scale, please rate your current sleepiness level:

1	Extremely alert	4	Fairly alert	7	Sleepy, but no effort to keep alert
2	Very alert	5	Neither alert or sleepy	8	Sleepy, some effort to keep alert
3	Alert	6	Some signs of sleepiness	9	Very sleepy, great effort to keep alert, fighting sleepiness

Before FD: ☐   After FD: ☐   After TD: ☐

During MD: ☐   After MD: ☐   After debriefing: ☐

Part C: Daytime Sleep Level

Based on followng scale, please rate your chance of sleeping or dozing during these activities:

0 = never	1 = slight	2 = moderate	3 = high

Sitting and reading ☐

Watching TV ☐

Sitting inactive in public place ☐

Being a passenger in a motor vehicle for an hour or more ☐

Lying down in the afternon ☐

Sitting and talking to someone ☐

Sitting quietly after lunch (no alcohol) ☐

Stopped for a few minutes in traffic while driving ☐

Sleep and Monotonous Driving Condition   Subject No. : _____
Effect in Driving Simulator/Driver Drowsiness Detection using Physiological Signals

Part D: Sleep Quality

Please state:
    Time you went to bed last night: _____   Time you woke up this morning: _____

Did you nap before coming here?   Yes/No   If yes, how long did you nap?   _____ minutes

The following questions relate to your usual sleep habits during the past month only. Your answers should indicate the most accurate reply for the majority of days and nights in the past month. Please answer all questions.

During the past month,
    When do you usually gone to bed at night?   _____ p.m.

    How long does it usually take you to fall asleep each night?   _____ minutes

    When do you usually wake up in the morning?   _____ a.m.

    How many hours of *actual* sleep did you get at night? (This may be   _____ hours
    different than the number of hours you spend in bed)

For the remaining questions, please check only one best response. Please answer all questions.

During the past month, how often do you have trouble sleeping because you:

	not during the past	less than once a	once or twice a	three or more times
Cannot sleep within 30 minutes	☐	☐	☐	☐
Wake up in the middle of the night or early morning	☐	☐	☐	☐
Have to get up to use the bathroom	☐	☐	☐	☐
Cannot breathe comfortably	☐	☐	☐	☐
Cough or snore loudly	☐	☐	☐	☐
Feel too cold	☐	☐	☐	☐
Feel too hot	☐	☐	☐	☐
Had bad dreams	☐	☐	☐	☐
Have pain	☐	☐	☐	☐

During the past month, how often do you

	not during the past	less than once a	once or twice a	three or more times
taken medicine (prescribed or over the counter) to help you sleep?	☐	☐	☐	☐
had trouble staying awake while driving, eating meals or engaging in social activity?	☐	☐	☐	☐

During the past month, how would you rate your overall sleep quality?
☐ very good   ☐ fairly good   ☐ fairly bad   ☐ very bad

APPENDIX 14 SUBJECT RESEARCH INFORMATION

RESEARCH INFORMATION

Research Title: **Mental Stress Evaluation Using Physiological Signals** (See Chapter 02: Mental Stress)

Researcher's Name: **

MMC Registration No.: **

INTRODUCTION

You are invited to take part voluntarily in a research study on mental stress evaluation.

Your participation in this study is expected to last up to 3 hours. Up to 60 subjects will be participating in this study.

PURPOSE OF THE STUDY

The purpose of this study is to determine your cognitive performance in terms of physiological markers.

It is also possible that information collected in this experiment will be used in future research.

QUALIFICATION TO PARTICIPATE

Requirements for participation in this study:
- Enrolled in UTP or USM
- Age from 18 to 25 years and ability to give consent
  You **cannot** participate in this study if:
- you do not give consent.
- you have any head injury or neurological disease like epilepsy, seizures, or migraine, or any other forms of psychological disorders.
- you are under any type of daily medication.
- you have any type of skin allergy.

STUDY PROCEDURES

Upon your arrival to the experiment room, you will be given this Research Information Form. If you agree to participate, you will have to sign a consent form. Your head will be measured to select the appropriate size of electrode cap. Two points will be marked on your forehead at 10% of the total distance from your anion to nasion. These marks are to locate the position of electrodes FP1 and FP2. The researcher in charge will explain to you about these terms.

The cap will be put on your head and two sponge donuts will be adhered on the marked points, so that the electrodes will not cause pain. Two electrodes will be connected to your earlobes. To make good connectivity, your ears will be abraded with Nurep paste and the electrodes will be filled with Nurep paste and the electrodes will be filled with Electro Gel. Electro Gel will also be injected in the Electro-Cap electrodes to make good connectivity with your scalp.

The impedance of all the electrodes will be measured and Electro-Cap electrodes may be abraded if they show high impedance. Two ECG sensors will be applied onto the second rib below the right and left shoulder blades. The application area will be cleaned and abraded to make good contact.

After all this setup, the experiment will start. The experiment flow is as follows:

Experiment 1:

1. 5 minutes rest time for habituation with the sensors
2. 5 minutes training
3. 10 minutes rest
4. 20 minutes stress condition
5. Fill in questionnaire
6. 10 minutes relaxation
7. 20 minutes control condition
8. Fill in questionnaire
9. 10 minutes recovery

Note: Every 20-minute condition is divided into 4 sessions. You are free to start every session; you can take a rest and relax your body if you want. But please make sure you are not blinking/rolling/moving your eyes, moving your body, stretching your muscles during the recording.

Experiment 2:

1. 5 minutes eyes-closed test
2. 5 minutes eyes-open test
3. 20 minutes 2D movies/games
4. Fill in questionnaire
5. 5 minutes eyes-open test
6. 20 minutes 3D movies/games with active glasses
7. Fill in questionnaire
8. 5 minutes eyes-open test
9. 20 minutes 3D movies/games with passive glasses
10. Fill in questionnaire
11. 5 minutes eyes-open test
12. 20 minutes 3D movies/games autostereoscopic monitor
13. Fill in questionnaire

Note: Every 20-minute session is divided into 3–4 minutes recording. After every 3–4 minutes, you will be given a break to take a rest and relax your body. But please make sure you are not blinking/rolling/moving your eyes, moving your body, or stretching your muscles.

RISKS

There exists the possibility of risk and discomfort occurring during the test that could include skin irritation, allergy, or tears in eyes. To minimize these conditions, you will be frequently asked by the experimenter if you are experiencing any discomfort and your electroencephalogram will be closely monitored.

REPORTING HEALTH EXPERIENCES

If you have any injury, bad effects, or any other unusual health experience during this study, make sure that you immediately tell the experimenter.

PARTICIPATION IN THE STUDY

Your taking part in this study is entirely voluntary. You may refuse to take part in the study or you may stop participation in the study at any time, without a penalty or loss of benefits to which you are otherwise entitled. During this 3-hour session, if you feel any discomfort or pain, or if you feel sleepy, tell the researcher in charge to stop recording and give you some rest. Your participation may also be stopped by the researcher in charge without your consent if you do not follow the instructions, blink/roll/move your eyes too much, or feel sleepy during the recording. However at the successful completion of the experiment, you will be given RM 50.00 to compensate your time spent.

QUESTIONS

If you have any questions about this study or your rights or regarding the Ethical Approval or any issue/problem related to this study, please contact:

CONFIDENTIAL

Your information will be kept confidential by the study staff and will not be made publicly available unless disclosure is required by law.

Data obtained from this study that does not identify you individually will be published for knowledge purposes. Your medical information may be held and processed on a computer.

By signing this consent form, you authorize the record review, information storage, and data transfer described above.

SIGNATURES

To be entered into the study, you or a legal representative must sign and date the signature page (see Appendix 2C).

RESEARCH INFORMATION

Research Title:	**Developing of EEG Based Biomarker for MDD** (See Chapter 03: Major Depressive Disorder)
Researcher's Name:	************************************
MMC Registration No.:	************************************

INTRODUCTION

You are invited to voluntarily take part in this research study for a duration of 4 weeks. During this period you will be treated with a type of medicine (an antidepressant) prescribed by a medical doctor at Hospital Universiti Sain Malaysia (HUSM). After you sign the consent form, demographic information will be collected by filling out a questionnaire. The venue for data collection will be at HUSM. Fig. A.1 summarizes recording sessions during the 4 weeks. A total of five (5) recording sessions are included: the first one is carried out before medication regarded as the baseline, and the other sessions will be performed during medication. In each session there will be two (2) types of recording: electrophysiological (EEG) and clinical assessment of disease severity using the BDI-II and HADS questionnaires.

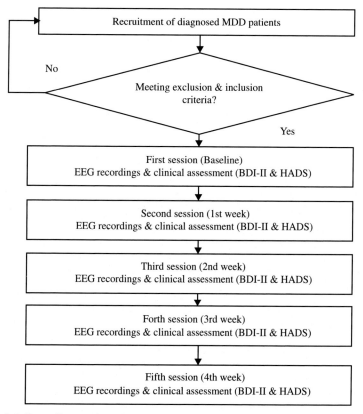

Figure A.1 Recording sessions.

Both the EEG and clinical assessment will be carried out on the same day. The section "Study Procedure" describes the recording details.

PURPOSE OF THE STUDY

Generally clinical doctors need to wait 4 weeks to observe outcomes of first treatment (improvement, response, remission) of MDD patients. Unfortunately, if the treatment has no or little effect, the medicine used needs to be changed. It means the further treatment will be delayed. It is necessary to develop a method to assist medical doctors early to select an effective medicine for these MDD patients during the treatment. The purpose of this study is to design a predictive biomarker (model) based on the information extracted from EEG data and clinical severity scores. This biomarker intends to assist doctors to predict treatment efficacy in a shorter period of time as compared to the clinical methods.

QUALIFICATION TO PARTICIPATE

Requirements for participation in this study:
- Written informed consent
- Patients with age 18–65 years
- Patients diagnosed MDD (DSM-IV)
  - Newly diagnosed (new cases)
  - Newly started (old cases)
    - Restarted on antidepressant (1 week washout)
    - Switched to new antidepressant

Participant who cannot participate in this study:
- Patients having psychotic, cognitive disorder
- Patients with any other drug abuse
- Pregnant patients
- Patients with epilepsy

STUDY PROCEDURE

1. EEG data collection

EEG data collection consists of four (4) steps seen in Fig. A.2. A total of 40 minutes is required.

Step 1 is to set up the experiment using a 24-channel wearable cap. The suitable cap will be selected by measuring your head size using a

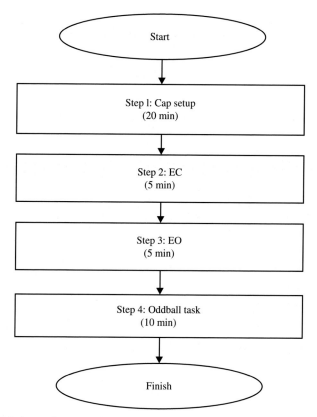

Fig. A.2 EEG data collection scheme.

head measuring tape. Proper setting up of the cap will be important for data quality. This process will take about 20 minutes;

Step 2 is the eyes-closed (EC) session: you are required to sit on a chair with eyes-closed and **not to fall asleep**. This will take about 5 minutes;

Step 3 is the eyes-open (EO) session: you are required to look at a fixation point ("**+**") on a computer screen in front of you with **minimal eye movement** and **blinking**. This requires nearly 5 minutes;

Step 4 is a visual 3-stimulus oddball task: you will be exposed to a random sequence of shapes on a computer screen. Only one (1) shape will be displayed at a time. There are a total of three (3) shapes (Fig. A.3):

Target (a blue circle) with 5.0 cm size;
Standard (a blue circle) with 4.5 cm size;
Distractor (a checkerboard) with 18.0 cm size.

Visual 3-Stimulus oddball task

Category	Stimulus	Component
Target (0.12)	5.0 cm	P3b (P300)
Distracter (0.12)	18.0 cm 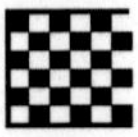	P3a
Standard (0.76)	4.5 cm	N1, P2, N2 (Sensory potentials)

Category=P3a/P3b stimulus type (probability). Stimulus=physical characteristics and width. Component= potentials produced for specific conditions. Blue circles were presented on light gray background and the checkerboard was composed of black and white checks approximately 1 cm square.

Fig. A.3 3-Stimulus visual oddball task.

You **must** respond to the **Target** shape by pressing the **SPACE** key on the keyboard, but **NO** action must be taken in response to other shapes. This process will take about 10 minutes.

2. Clinical assessment using BDI-II and HADS

The questionnaire-based forms will be filled out by a medical doctor after asking questions.

RISKS

There exists the possibility of discomfort during the study that may include skin irritation or strain/tears in eyes. During the study you are required to report to research staff if you are experiencing any discomfort. If this is the case, the recording will be terminated. Your EEG recordings will be closely monitored.

REPORTING HEALTH EXPERIENCES

It is your responsibility to inform research staff about health experiences such as discomfort during the study and/or previous injury, particularly head injury. If this is the case, the recording will be terminated.

PARTICIPATION IN THE STUDY

Your participation in the whole study is entirely voluntary with reward.

POSSIBLE BENEFITS

The results of this study will be used for future academic and research purposes and may also be made publicly available, which may have financial implications. However, the identity of the subject will be kept confidential.

QUESTIONS

If you have any questions about this study or your rights or regarding the ethical approval or any issue/problem related to this study, please contact:

CONFIDENTIALITY

Your identity will be kept confidential and will not be made publicly available unless disclosure is required by law.

Data obtained from this study that does not identify you individually will be published for academic and research purposes and for publicly available databases.

Your medical information may be held and processed on a computer.

By signing this consent form, you authorize the record review, information storage, and data transfer described above.

SIGNATURES

To be entered into the study, you or a legal representative must sign and date the signature page (see Appendix 2C).

RESEARCH INFORMATION

Research Title: **Memory Retention and Recall Processes for 3D Contents** (See Chapter 07: 2D and 3D Educational Contents)

Researcher's Name: ***

INTRODUCTION

You are invited to take part voluntarily in a research study of memory retention and recall processes using 2D and 3D contents (animation, objects, and images).

This study is comprised of four sessions: the first session will take up to 2 hours. So your participation in this study is expected to last within 2 hours in this session, and approximately less than 2 hours for each of the remaining sessions; each session will be conducted after a 2-month period.

PURPOSE OF THE STUDY

The purpose of this study is to determine the effects of 3D educational tools on learning, retention, and retrieval of information as compared to 2D educational tools. You will learn from either 2D contents or 3D contents and then will recall the learned contents through prescribed procedure.

QUALIFICATION TO PARTICIPATE

The member of this study staff has discussed with you the requirements for participation in this study. It is important that you are completely truthful with the staff about your health history. You should not participate in this study if you do not meet all qualifications.

Some of the requirements to be in this study are:
- You must be between 18 and 28 years old
- You must be physically and mentally healthy
  You cannot participate in this study if:
- You fail to provide written consent
- You fail to meet the requirements asked in the screening questionnaire

STUDY PROCEDURES

This experiment consists of four sessions. In the first session, when you arrive at the experiment room, you will be asked to first complete a questionnaire asking some questions about health-related issues and any medications you may be taking. When it is ensured that you do not have any health issues that may affect the experiment, you will be given this informed consent form. If you agree to participate, please provide your consent by signing the consent form. After providing consent, you will be asked to complete an intelligence test. Upon completion, an electrode cap will be placed on your head. The cap is snug fitting, and we will need to squirt some gel onto each electrode to help us make good measurements of your brain waves. It will take about 15–20 minutes to get the cap fitted properly.

During brain signal recording, you will be asked to perform two types of memory tasks. In the first type of task, you will be asked to do a Sternberg task and N–back task that will require you to observe and remember the shapes (either 2D shape or 3D shape) displayed on screen and respond to a target shape, to assess the previously observed shapes. In the second type of task, you will be asked to watch a 3D/2D based animation about a general topic from biology, physics, or chemistry that will be assessed via a recall task after 2 months in the later sessions. Both types of task will last approximately 30 minutes, and you will be given few-minute breaks at regular intervals to take rest. After you have completed the memory tasks, you will be asked to fill out a feedback questionnaire about the environment (2D or 3D) in which you have observed and remembered objects, and about your perception. Participation will take approximately 2 hours of your time in the first session. The following sessions (2nd, 3rd, and 4th sessions) will be conducted after a delay of 2 months. In the 2nd, 3rd, and 4th sessions, you have to perform a retrieval task, in which you retrieve the contents you have observed in the first session (see Table A.2 for session activities).

Table A.2 Session wise activities

Session no.	Delay period	Time duration approx.	Tasks	Brain signal recording
1st session	0	Up to 2 hours	Consent form Screening questionnaire IQ test Memory tasks for STM/WM 3D/2D Animation contents for LTM Feedback questionnaire	EEG data recording during memory tasks and at rest state
2nd session	2 months	Up to 1 hour	Memory retrieval task about 3D/2D animation contents	EEG data recording
3rd session	2 months	Up to 1 hour	Memory retrieval task about 3D/2D animation contents	EEG data recording
4th session	2 months	Up to 1 hour	Memory retrieval task about 3D/2D animation contents	EEG data recording

RISKS

While EEG measurements have been used widely, including in neuropsychological studies, there have been no reports of severe accidents specific to EEG. But there is the possibility of discomfort or the risk of skin irritation or allergy during the test. To check for such discomfort, you will be frequently asked by the experimenter if you feel uncomfortable and your electroencephalogram will be closely monitored.

REPORTING HEALTH EXPERIENCES

If you have any problem or feel uncomfortable during this study, please inform the experimenter immediately.

PARTICIPATION IN THE STUDY

Your taking part in this study is entirely voluntary. You may terminate or refuse to continue your participation in the study at any time without any penalty. During the whole experiment session, if you feel any discomfort or pain, please tell the experimenter to stop recording and allow you to rest or take a short break. In the case where you do not comply with the experimental procedure, your participation may be stopped by the experimenter.

POSSIBLE BENEFITS

This research study will investigate the effects of 2D versus 3D contents on memory retention and recall processes. The results of this study will be used for future academic and research purposes.

QUESTIONS

If you have any questions regarding the Ethical Approval or any issue/problem related to this study, please contact:

CONFIDENTIALITY

Your data will be kept confidential by the experimenter and will not be made publicly available unless disclosure is required by law.

Data obtained from this study that does not identify you individually will be published for academic and research purposes only.

By signing this consent form, you authorize the record review, information storage, and data transfer described above.

SIGNATURES

To become a participant in this study, you have to sign the attached consent and give it to the experimenter (see Appendix 2C).

By signing this consent form, you authorize the record review, information storage, and data transfer described above.

RESEARCH INFORMATION

Research Title:	**Analyzing Effects of 3D Video Games Contents Using Electroencephalography (EEG)** (See Chapter 9: 3D Video Games)
Researcher's Name:	**************************************

INTRODUCTION

You are invited to take part voluntarily in a research study of the effects of video games contents using 2D and 3D contents (animation, objects, and images).

This study comprised of three sessions. The first session will take about 30 minutes, during which you need to complete a questionnaire before taking part in the experiments. The second session will take up to 1 hour; this session is for you to practice the game first before the real session. The third session will take up to 2 hours. So your participation in this study is expected to last within 2 hours in this session. All sessions will take around 2 days of completion for each participant.

PURPOSE OF THE STUDY

The purpose of the present study is to analyze the effects of exposure to different 3D video games contents compared to 2D video games on brain signal activities. You will learn from either 2D contents or 3D contents and then will recall the learned contents through the prescribed procedure.

QUALIFICATION TO PARTICIPATE

A member of this study staff has discussed with you the requirements for participation in this study. It is important that you are completely truthful with the staff about your health history. You should not participate in this study if you do not meet all qualifications.

Some of the requirements to be in this study are:

- You must be between 18 and 28 years old
- You must be physically and mentally healthy
  You cannot participate in this study if:
- You fail to provide written consent
- You fail to meet the requirements asked in the screening questionnaire

STUDY PROCEDURES

This experiment consists of three sessions. In the first session, you will be given a questionnaire asking some questions about health-related issues and your experiences playing video games. When it is ensured that you do not have any health issues that may affect the experiment and that you fulfill the requirements, you will be given this informed consent form. If you agree to participate, please provide your consent by signing the consent form. After providing consent, you will be asked to come for the second session.

For the second session, you will be asked to practice playing violent video games so that you will be familiar with the game. You will be playing in 2D and 3D alternately. This session will take about 1 hour practice for each participant. After complete the practice session, you are needed to come back for the third session the next day. Finally, for the third session, an electrode cap will be placed on your head. The cap is snug fitting, and we will need to squirt some gel onto each electrode to help us make good measurements of your brain waves. It will take about 15–20 minutes to get the cap fitted properly.

During brain signal recording, you will be asked to perform four tasks. In the first task, you will be ask to stare at a cross "X" with white background paper for 5 minutes and blink your eyes within 1 minute intervals. For the second 5 minutes, you are required to stare the cross "X" right and left alternately within 1 minute to measure the eye movement artifacts. The first 10 minutes recording is to analyze the electroencephalography (EEG) artifacts. For the second task, you will be given 20 minutes to practice the game in 2D. During this time, you are required to already know how to play the game. In the third task, you will play the games in 2D for

Table A.3 Session wise activities

Session no.	Time duration approx.	Tasks	Brain signal recording
1st session	30 minutes	Screening questionnaire, consent form	No data recording
2nd session	60 minutes	Practice playing the violence video game in 2D and 3D	No data recording
3rd session	100 minutes	Calibration process, play the violence video game in 2D and 3D	EEG data recording

30 minutes. The brain signal will be recorded during the last 5 minutes of your play. Finally, for the fourth task, you will play the games in 3D for 30 minutes and your brain signal will be recorded during the last 5 minutes of your play. All tasks will last approximately 100 minutes, and you will be given 5-minute breaks at regular intervals to take a rest. After you have completed the tasks, you will be asked to fill out a feedback questionnaire about the effects on your health. Participation will take approximately 2 days of your time in this experiment (see Table A.3 for session activities).

RISKS

While EEG measurements have been used widely, including in neuropsychological studies, there have been no reports of severe accidents specific to EEG. But there is the possibility of discomfort or the risk of skin irritation or allergy during the test. To check for such discomfort, you will be frequently asked by the experimenter if you feel uncomfortable and your electroencephalogram will be closely monitored.

REPORTING HEALTH EXPERIENCES

If you have any problem or feel uncomfortable during this study, please inform the experimenter immediately.

PARTICIPATION IN THE STUDY

Your taking part in this study is entirely voluntary. You may terminate or refuse to continue your participation in the study at any time without any penalty. During the whole experiment session, if you feel any discomfort or pain, please tell the experimenter to stop recording and allow you to rest or take a short break. In the case where you do not comply with the experimental procedure, your participation may be stopped by the experimenter.

POSSIBLE BENEFITS

This research study will investigate the effects of 2D versus 3D contents of video games on the human brain by using EEG. The results of this study will be used in future academic and research purposes and may also be made publicly available, which may have financial implications. However, the identity of the subject will be kept confidential.

QUESTIONS

If you have any questions regarding the Ethical Approval or any issue/problem related to this study, please contact:

CONFIDENTIALITY

Your identity will be kept confidential and will not be made publicly available unless disclosure is required by law.

Data obtained from this study that does not identify you individually will be published for academic and research purposes and for publicly available databases.

By signing this consent form, you authorize the record review, information storage, and data transfer described above.

SIGNATURES

To become participant of this study you have to sign the attached consent and give it to the experimenter (see Appendix 2C).

By signing this consent form, you authorize the record review, information storage, and data transfer described above.

RESEARCH INFORMATION

Research Title:	**Visually Induced Motion Sickness for 3D** (See Chapter 10: Visually Induced Motion Sickness)
Researcher's Name:	************************************
MMC Registration No.:	************************************

INTRODUCTION

You are invited to take part voluntarily in a research study of visually induced motion sickness from 3D movies and images.

Your participation in this study is expected to last up to 3 hours. Up to 30 subjects will be participating in this study.

PURPOSE OF THE STUDY

The purpose of this study is to determine how your brain perceives information presented in 3D compared to 2D in terms of:
- Visually induced motion sickness (VIMS)
- Visual strain
- Understanding of displayed contents

It is also possible that information collected in this experiment will be used in future research.

QUALIFICATION TO PARTICIPATE

Requirements for participation in this study:
- Enrolled in a university program.
- Age from 18 to 40 years and ability to give consent.
  You cannot participate in this study if:
- You do not give consent.
- You have any head injury or neurological disease like epilepsy, seizures, and migraine, or any other form of psychological disorder.
- You have any eye disease, have had eye surgery, or have any history of eye injury or trauma.
- You are under any type of daily medication.
- You have any type of skin allergy.

STUDY PROCEDURES

Upon your arrival to the experiment room, you will be given this research information form. If you agree to participate, you will have to sign a consent form. Your head will be measured for placement of an electrode cap. Two points will be marked on your forehead at the center of your head for exact placement of the cap.

The impedance of all the electrodes will be measured and Electro-Cap electrodes may be abraded if they show high impedance. Two ECG sensors will be applied onto the second rib below the right and left shoulder blades. The application area will be cleaned and abraded to make good contact.

Two Velcro straps will be fit snugly around your forefinger and middle finger to measure your skin conductance. The electrode leads will be connected with these straps.

Eye gaze recording will be done through an eye tracking device. You will be asked to report about sickness level continuously on a sickness scale. This will be done by an input key from an input device. Reporting will be on a regular interval of 1 minute.

After all this setup, the experiment will start. The experiment flow is as follows:

1. 5 minutes eyes–closed test
2. 5 minutes eyes–open test
3. 10 minutes movie viewing
4. Fill in questionnaire

RISKS

There exists the possibility of risk and discomfort occurring during the test that could include skin irritation, allergy, or tears in eyes. To minimize these conditions, you will be frequently asked by the experimenter if you are experiencing any discomfort and your electroencephalogram will be closely monitored.

REPORTING HEALTH EXPERIENCES

If you have any injury, bad effect, or any other unusual health experience during this study, make sure that you immediately tell the experimenter.

PARTICIPATION IN THE STUDY

Your taking part in this study is entirely voluntary. You may refuse to take part in the study or you may stop participation in the study at any time, without a penalty or loss of benefits to which you are otherwise entitled. During this 3-hour session, if you feel any discomfort or pain, or if you feel sleepy, tell the researcher in charge to stop recording and give you some rest. Your participation may also be stopped by the researcher in charge without your consent if you do not follow the instructions, blink/roll/move your eyes too much, or feel sleepy during the recording. In this case you will be given RM 20.00 to compensate your spent time. If you successfully complete the whole experiment then you will be given RM 50.00 to compensate your spent time.

QUESTIONS

If you have any questions about this study or your rights regarding the Ethical Approval or any issue/problem related to this study, please contact:

CONFIDENTIALITY

Your information will be kept confidential by the study staff and will not be made publicly available unless disclosure is required by law.

Data obtained from this study that does not identify you individually will be published for knowledge purposes.

Your medical information may be held and processed on a computer.

By signing this consent form, you authorize the record review, information storage, and data transfer described above.

SIGNATURES

To be entered into the study, you or a legal representative must sign and date the signature page (see Appendix 2C).

REFERENCES

1. Dupont W.D., Plummer W.D. *PS: Power and sample size calculation.* Available from: http://biostat.mc.vanderbilt.edu/wiki/Main/PowerSampleSize; 2011.
2. Lal SKL. *The* psychophysiology of driver fatigue/drowsinees: PHD, Department of Health Sciences, University of Technology Sydney (UTS); 2001.
3. Patel M, Lal S, Kavanagh D, Rossiter P. Applying neural network analysis on heart rate variability data to assess driver fatigue. Exp Syst Appl. 2011;38:7235–7242.
4. Cantero JL, Atienza M, Salas RM, Gómez CM. Alpha EEG coherence in different brain states: an electrophysiological index of the arousal level in human subjects. Neurosci Lett 1999;271:167–170.

GLOSSARY

Alternative hypothesis The alternative hypothesis is the hypothesis that sample observations are influenced by some nonrandom cause. It is the hypothesis to be accepted if the null hypothesis is rejected.

A/D accuracy Accuracy specifies the maximum difference between the actual analog values compared with the value measured. If the feed a 2.5 V signal to an A/D input, the accuracy is a measure of how closely the A/D indicates the applied voltage is actually 2.5 V.

A/D resolution Resolution defines the smallest increment of change that can be detected in an analog measurement. If the A/D input range of 0 to +10 V with 12-bit resolution, then the range of 10 V is divided into 12 bits, or 4096 divisions. Therefore, a 1-bit change from the A/D input corresponds to a difference of 0.00244 V (10 V/4096 counts). Increasing the bits of precision that is returned by the A/D input will increase the resolution by decreasing each count of the A/D input.

Accommodation It is the process by which the human eye changes optical power to maintain a clear image or focus on an object as its distance varies. The act of adjustment of the eye for seeing objects at various distances. This is accomplished by the ciliary muscle, which controls the lens of the eye, allowing it to flatten or thicken as is needed for distant or near vision.

Active shutter It is a kind of 3D technology that uses battery-operated shutter glasses that do as their name describes: they rapidly shutter open and closed. This, in theory, means the information meant for your left eye is blocked from your right eye by a closed (opaque) shutter.

Alcohol abusers Individuals who abuse alcohol. Alcoholism is the most severe form of problem drinking. Alcoholism involves all the symptoms of alcohol abuse, but it also involves another element: physical dependence on alcohol.

Amplifier An amplifier is an electronic device that increases the voltage, current, or power of a signal. In EEG, the voltage of neurons is very small, which is required to be amplified.

Amplifier bandwidth The range of signal frequencies over which an amplifier is capable of undistorted or unattenuated transmission.

Antidepressant Medicine that is used in the treatment of mood disorders known as depression.

Artifacts In EEG recordings, recorded activity that is not of cerebral origin is called an artifact. In other words, the unwanted components of a signal are the artifacts.

Averaged epochs The outcome of the averaging of a number of epochs that are time-locked to similar events.

Averaged ERP The preprocessed ERP after averaging all the good trials is known as averaged ERP signal.

Averaged reference The EEG reference in which an average of all the EEG channels is used as a reference.

Averaging The combination of EEG segments from multiple trials or events or epochs in order to improve the EEG SNR (signal-to-noise ratio).

Baseline In ERP signals, a baseline signal is the segment of the signal present before the events of interest.

Baseline EEG In EEG signals, eyes open and eyes closed are known as the baseline EEG.

BDI-II Beck Depression Inventory-II (BDI-II) is a tool widely used as an indicator of the severity of depression.

Behavioral data The type of data recorded during an experiment related to the behavior of participants, such as correct answer, reaction time, false responses, etc.

BESA This is an EEG analysis software program, specializing in source analysis for EEG.

Binocular parallax The difference in the angles formed by the lines of sight to two objects situated at different distances from the eyes; a factor in the visual perception of depth.

Binocular vision Vision using two eyes with overlapping fields of view, allowing good perception of depth.

Biofeedback EEG biofeedback is a learning strategy that enables persons to alter their brain waves. When information about a person's own brain wave characteristics is made available to him, he or she can learn to change them.

Bipolar Bipolar means that there are two electrodes per one channel, so each channel has a reference electrode.

Block A time interval that possesses trials from one condition.

Blocked design The separation of experimental conditions into separate distinct blocks, so that the dependent variable could be compared in each block condition.

BOLD Blood-oxygen-level dependent imaging is a method used in functional magnetic resonance imaging (fMRI) to observe different areas of the brain or other organs that are found to be active at any given time.

Brain oscillations Also called neural oscillations, this term refers to the rhythmic and/or repetitive electrical activity generated spontaneously and in response to stimuli by neural tissue in the central nervous system. The importance of brain oscillations in sensory–cognitive processes has become increasingly evident

BrainMaster Discovery It is a EEG data acquisition software used with the BrainMaster amplifier, developed by Applied Neuroscience, Inc.

CAR (common average reference) It is the average of all the electrodes' electrical activity to be used as reference for each EEG electrode.

Categorial variable A variable that can take one of several discrete values.

Central executive It is an important component of the working memory model developed by Baddeley and Hitch in 1974. Drives the whole system (e.g., the boss of working memory) and allocates data to the subsystems (visuospatial sketchpad and phonological loop). It also deals with cognitive tasks such as mental arithmetic and problem solving.

Channel bandwidth A channel is the medium through which EEG is recorded from the brain over the scalp via EEG amplifier. Channel bandwidth is the frequency range that constitutes the channel.

Code division multiple access (CDMA) CDMA refers to any of several protocols used in second-generation (2G) and third-generation (3G) wireless communications. As the term implies, CDMA is a form of multiplexing, which allows numerous signals to occupy a single transmission channel, optimizing the use of available bandwidth. The technology is used in ultrahigh-frequency (UHF) cellular telephone systems in the 800-MHz and 1.9-GHz bands.

Cognitive disorder Any disorder that significantly impairs the cognitive function (learning, memory, perception, and problem solving, including amnesia, dementia, and delirium) of an individual to the point where normal functioning in society is impossible without treatment.

Cognitive distraction Cognitive distraction is simply another way to describe driver inattention, i.e., not keeping your eyes and mind on the road. Cognitive distraction occurs when an individual's focus is not directly on the act of driving and his/her mind "wanders."

Computational techniques The mathematical methods used for analysis of EEG to differentiate between groups or conditions.

Conditions (levels) More than one value of the independent variable.

Confounding factor Any property that covaries with the independent variable of the conducted experiment and could be separated from the independent variable using a different experiment design.

Continuous variable A variable that can take any value within a given range.

Contralateral delay activity (CDA) This is a negative slow wave sensitive to the number of objects maintained in visual working memory.

Control block A block that contains trials of the control condition.

Control condition It is also called baseline condition or nonexperimental condition, because it provides a standard to which the experimental condition can be compared.

Convergence The ability of the eyes to move and work as a team.

Data acquisition The process of measuring the brain electrical activity via EEG equipment.

DC amplifier It is a kind of amplifier in which the output of one stage of the amplifier is coupled to the input of the next stage. It is used for EEG recording.

Dependent variable (DV) Quantities that are measured or tested by the experimenter to find the effects of the independent variables.

Depth perception The ability to perceive the relative distance of objects in one's visual field.

Detection Identification of whether or not an EEG activity within a certain condition changes in response to the experimental manipulation.

Disparity The condition of being unequal or totally different. The word is used mainly to refer to noncorresponding points in the retina.

Dizziness It is classified into three categories: vertigo, syncope, and nonsyncope nonvertigo. Each category has a characteristic set of symptoms, all related to the sense of balance. In general, syncope is defined by a brief loss of consciousness (fainting) or by dimmed vision and feeling uncoordinated, confused, and lightheaded. Many people experience a sensation like syncope when they stand up too fast. Vertigo is the feeling that either the individual or the surroundings are spinning. This sensation is like being on a spinning amusement park ride. Individuals with nonsyncope nonvertigo dizziness feel as though they cannot keep their balance. This feeling may become worse with movement.

Driving simulator Driving simulators are technologies used for entertainment as well as in training of driver's education courses taught in educational institutions and private businesses.

Drowsiness Sleep-deprived driving also known as tired driving, drowsy driving, or fatigued driving is the operation of a motor vehicle while being cognitively impaired by a lack of sleep.

DSM-IV The *Diagnostic and Statistical Manual of Mental Disorders*, published by the American Psychiatric Association, offers a common language and standard criteria for the classification of mental disorders. The fourth edition (DSM-IV) covers all the mental disorders for both children and adults.

EDF European data format (EDF) is a file format normally used to store EEG data.

EEG Stands for electroencephalography. It is the measurement of the electrical potential of the brain cortical activity usually recorded via electrodes placed on the surface of the scalp.

EEG references Electric potentials are only defined with respect to a reference electrode, i.e., an arbitrarily chosen "zero level."

Effect size It is a simple way of quantifying the difference between two groups that has many advantages over the use of tests of statistical significance alone. It emphasizes the size of the difference rather than confounding this with sample size.

EGI Electrical Geodesics, Inc. (EGI) is a US manufacturing company of EEG high-density systems. The EGI Net Amp with Net Station software is the main EEG product of the company.

Electrocardiogram (ECG) An electrocardiogram (ECG) is a technique that can be used to check the heart's rhythm and electrical activity.

Electrode An electrode is an electrical conductor used to make contact with the scalp of the participant.

Electrolyte A liquid or gel that contains ions and can be decomposed by electrolysis. In EEG recording, it is used to increase conductivity and record good signals.

Electromyogram (EMG) Electromyography (EMG) is a diagnostic procedure to assess the health of muscles and the nerve cells that control them (motor neurons). It measures the electrical activity of muscles at rest and during contraction.

Electrooculogram (EOG) This measures the corneoretinal standing potential that exists between the front and the back of the human eye.

EM radiation Electromagnetic radiation is energy that is propagated through free space or through a material medium in the form of electromagnetic waves, such as radio waves, visible light, and gamma rays. The term also refers to the emission and transmission of such radiant energy.

Empirical Based on experiment rather than theory.

Encoding Encoding is the initial important process of creating new memories. It allows the perceived item of interest to be converted into a construct that can be stored within the brain, and then recalled later from short-term or long-term memory. Encoding is a biological event beginning with perception through the senses.

Enobio It is an EEG recording machine developed by neuroelectrics.

Epileptic disorder Epilepsy is a brain disorder in which clusters of nerve cells, or neurons, in the brain sometimes signal abnormally, causing strange sensations, emotions, and behavior, or sometimes convulsions, muscle spasms, and loss of consciousness.

Epileptogenic tissues The brain tissues in which the epilepsy is developed.

Epoch A time segment extracted from a continuous EEG usually corresponding to the period in time surrounding an event of interest.

E-Prime Software used to control the stimuli presentation in an experiment.

Ergonomic The process of designing or arranging workplaces, products, and systems so that they fit the people who use them.

Ethical principles The rules associated with ethics.

Ethics The moral principles that govern a person's or group's behavior.

Ethics approval An approval of conducting experimental research with animal or human subjects from a standard specialized authorized body.

Ethics committee The authorized body or group of experts who can evaluate a study for conducting experimental research.

Event It is also called a trial. A single instance of the experimental manipulation.

Event-related design The presentation of discrete and short duration events with randomizable timing and order.

Event-related potentials (ERP) Electrical changes in the brain associated with sensory or cognitive events in time-lock EEG.

Events synchronization Events occurring at the same time.

Experiment The controlled test of a hypothesis. Experiments manipulate one or more independent variables, measure one or more dependent variables, and evaluate measurements using statistical significance.

Experiment design The step-by-step organization of an experiment to conduct effect testing of the research hypothesis.

Experimental condition It is also known as task condition, because it contains the stimuli or task relevant to the research hypothesis.

Eye strain The term eye strain is frequently used by people to describe a group of symptoms that are related to use of the eyes. Eye strain is a symptom, not an eye disease. Eye strain occurs when your eyes get tired from intense use, such as when driving a car for extended periods, reading, or working at a computer.

Eye tracking The process of measuring either the point of gaze (where one is looking) or the motion of the eye relative to the head.

Feature extraction Extracting useful information from EEG signals using statistical or computational methods.

Feedback Information about reactions to an event or stimuli in experiment by the participants.

Filtering A filter is a function or process that retains some part of interest in a signal and removes unwanted components from a signal. In EEG signal processing, filtering is the removal of the very low frequency component and very high frequency component, e.g., 0.5–30.0 Hz.

Fixation In visual research experiment, this is the maintaining of the visual gaze on a single location. It is also used in EEG experiments where visual stimuli are involved.

Fluid intelligence The general ability to think abstractly, reason, identify patterns, solve problems, and discern relationships.

Gastrointestinal distress Gastroparesis is a medical term that means decreased gut motility or delayed emptying of the stomach and small intestines.

Global system for mobile communications (GSM) GSM is a digital mobile telephony system that is widely used in Europe and other parts of the world. It uses a variation of time division multiple access (TDMA) and digitizes and compresses data, then sends it down a channel with two other streams of user data, each in its own time slot. It operates at either the 900 MHz or 1800 MHz frequency band.

GUI Graphic user interface (GUI) is a terminology of computer science and a type of user interface that allows users to interact with electronic devices through graphical icons and visual indicators, such as secondary notation, instead of text-based user interfaces, typed command labels, or text navigation.

HADS Hospital Anxiety and Depression Scale (HADS) is a tool used to diagnose mental disorders such as depression and anxiety.

Headaches A feeling of pain in the head due to watching visual stimuli such as 3D contents.

Head-mounted displays (HMDs) Head-mounted displays (HMDs) are small displays or projection technology integrated into eyeglasses or mounted on a helmet or hat.

Heart rate variability (HRV) The physiological phenomenon of variation in the time interval between heartbeats.

High-density EEG with large number of channels.

HUSM Hospital University Sains Malaysia (HUSM).

Hyperopia Hyperopia (farsightedness) is the condition of the eye in which incoming rays of light reach the retina before they converge into a focused image.

IBM IBM-International Business Machines Corporation is a multinational technology company headquartered at New York, United States.

ICA Independent component analysis (ICA) is a computational method for separating a multivariate signal into additive subcomponents.

Illusion Something that is likely to be wrongly perceived or interpreted by the senses. In 3D technology, depth illusion is created for the viewers.

Impedance The resistance to current flow at certain electrode is measured in ohms, known as impedance.

Impule A short duration response of the neurons, or a single input to a system.

Independent variable (IV) Variable that is hypothesized in a scientific experiment to cause changes in the dependent variable.

Informed consent A permission granted with the knowledge of the possible consequences, typically that which is given by a patient to a doctor for treatment with full knowledge of the possible risks and benefits.

Inion The projecting part of the occipital bone at the base of the skull.

Interstimulus interval (ISI) The time between the offset of one stimulus and the onset of the next stimulus or separation in time between successive stimuli.

Intertrial interval (ITI) An intertrial interval (ITI) is the time between separate trials (conditioning by presentation of stimuli) in behaviorist learning research. The ITI is usually measured at the beginning of a trial and lasts until the beginning of the following trial.

Intervention A health intervention is an effort that promotes behavior that improves mental and physical health, or discourages or reframes those with health risks.

***Killzone 3* game** *Killzone 3* is a 2011 first-person shooter video game for the PlayStation 3, developed by Guerrilla Games and published by Sony Computer Entertainment.

Line noise A term that describes the disruption that can occur in EEG data recording or data transmissions through the interference of stray electromagnetic signals.

Long-term memory The capacity of retaining a large amount of information in mind for a long time.

Low density EEG with few channels.

Major depressive disorder A mental disorder, also known as depression or major depression, characterized by at least 2 weeks of low mood that is present across most situations.

Matching pursuit technique This is a sparse approximation algorithm that involves finding the "best matching" projections of multidimensional data onto the span of an overcomplete, i.e., redundant, dictionary D. It finds a suboptimal solution to the problem of an adaptive approximation of a signal in a redundant set (dictionary) of functions. Commonly used with dictionaries of Gabor functions, it offers several advantages in time–frequency analysis of signals, in particular EEG/MEG.

MEG Magnetoencephalogram (MEG) is a functional neuroimaging technique used to measure the magnetic fields generated by neuronal activity of the brain.

Memorization The process of creating new memories and transforming new information into memory storage.

Mental arithmetic task An experimental task in which arithmetic problems are presented as stimuli and participants have to mentally calculate the solution and respond.

Mental arithmetic task condition Experimental condition in which participants have to perform the mental arithmetic task.

Mental disorder Mental illness, also known as psychiatric disorder, e.g., depression, stress, anxiety, dementia, etc.

Mental process The term used to describe all the processes of mind, such as thinking, problem solving, memory, attention, information processing, as a whole.

Mental stress A state of mental tension and worry caused by problems in a person's life, work, etc.; something that causes strong feelings of worry or anxiety.

Migraine A familial, recurrent syndrome characterized usually by unilateral head pain, accompanied by various focal disturbances of the nervous system, particularly in regard to visual phenomenon, such as scintillating scotomas.

Mild psychological stress A kind of stress that is not severe.

Montage The configuration of EEG electrode placement during recording of EEG signals in an experiment.

Montreal Imaging Stress Task An experimental task that contains a series of mental arithmetic challenges used to assess psychological stress in humans.

Motion parallax Motion parallax is a monocular depth cue in which we view objects that are closer to us as moving faster than objects that are further away from us.

Multimedia tools Multimedia tools include a combination of different audio and visual content.

Myopia Myopia is the medical term for nearsightedness. People with myopia see objects more clearly when they are close to the eye, while distant objects appear blurred or fuzzy. Reading and close-up work may be clear, but distance vision is blurry.

Nasion The point of intersection of the frontal bone and two nasal bones of the human skull.

Nausea Nausea is an uneasiness of the stomach that often comes before vomiting.

Neurofeedback A type of biofeedback that uses real-time displays of brain activity, most commonly electroencephalography (EEG), to teach self-regulation of brain function.

Neuroguide A qEEG analysis software developed by Applied Neuroscience, Inc.

Nonaveraged ERP Nonaveraged, single-trial, or continuous EEG is the types of nonaveraged data.

Nonrapid eye movement (NREM) NREM (nonrapid eye movement) sleep is dreamless sleep. During NREM, the brain waves on the electroencephalographic (EEG) recording are typically slow and of high voltage, the breathing and heart rate are slow and regular, the blood pressure is low, and the sleeper is relatively still. NREM sleep is divided into four stages of increasing depth leading to REM sleep.

Null hypothesis The hypothesis states that there is no significant difference between specified populations, any observed difference being due to sampling or experimental error.

Null-task block Also called baseline block, because there are no task requirements for the participant.

Objective measures Those facts that are observable and measurable by the experimenter.

Oddball paradigm An experimental design used within event-related potential (ERP) research, where presentations of sequences of repetitive audio/visual stimuli are infrequently interrupted by a deviant stimulus.

P200 The ERP peak appearing at 200 milliseconds is known as P200 or P2.

P3 amplitude The amplitude of the P300 component appear in after 300 milliseconds in an ERP signal. It is measured in microvolts.

P3 latency The time from the stimulus onset to the point where the P300 peak appears.

P300 The P300 wave is a positive deflection in the human event-related potential. It is most commonly elicited in an oddball paradigm when a subject detects an occasional "target" stimulus in a regular train of standard stimuli. The P300 wave only occurs if the subject is actively engaged in the task of detecting the targets.

Passive polarized A kind of 3D system that uses polarization glasses to create the illusion of three-dimensional hardware-based product to facilitate 3D content creation.

Phonological loop The phonological loop is the part of working memory that deals with spoken and written material. It can be used to remember a phone number. It consists of two parts: the phonological store (inner ear) and the articulatory control process (inner voice). The former is linked to speech perception and holds information in speech-based form (i.e., spoken words) for 1–2 seconds; the latter is linked to speech production. Used to rehearse and store verbal information from the phonological store.

Physical stress Physical stress is a physical reaction of the body to various triggers. The pain experienced after surgery is an example of physical stress.

Physiological data Physiological data means recordings of brain activity (EEG), ECG, EMG, blood pressure, skin conductance, etc.

Polygraphic Input Box The Polygraph Input Box (PIB) is EGI's physiological measurement system. It allows the simultaneous measurement of peripheral nervous system activity and EEG. The PIB includes seven bipolar channel inputs for the measurement of electrocardiogram (ECG), electromyogram (EMG), respiration (effort, temperature, and pressure), and body position.

Population All the individuals or units that meet the selection criteria for a group to be studied.

Presbyopia The term presbyopia means "old eye" and is a vision condition involving the loss of the eye's ability to focus on close objects.

PSS questionnaire The perceived stress scale (PSS) is a psychological instrument for measuring the perception of stress.

Psychiatrist A physician who specializes in the diagnosis and treatment of behavioral abnormalities and mental diseases.

Psychotic A person suffering from a psychosis. Psychosis is a mental health problem that causes people to perceive or interpret things differently from those around them.

Radio frequency (RF) Radio frequency (RF) is any of the electromagnetic wave frequencies that lie in the range extending from around 3 kHz to 300 GHz, including those frequencies used for communications or radar signals. RF usually refers to electrical rather than mechanical oscillations. When an RF current is supplied to an antenna, an electromagnetic field is created that then is able to propagate through space. Many wireless technologies are based on RF field propagation.

Rapid eye movement (REM) REM sleep is when dreams occur. We have 3–5 REM periods per night. They occur at intervals of 1–2 hours apart and are quite variable in length, ranging from 5 minutes to over an hour. REM sleep is characterized by rapid, low-voltage brain waves, irregular breathing and heart rate, and involuntary muscle jerks.

Reaction time Reaction time is a measure of the quickness an organism responds to some sort of stimulus OR it is the elapsed time between the presentation of a sensory stimulus and the subsequent behavioral response.

Recruitment Hiring human subjects to participate in experiment.

Referential The referential montage means that there is a common reference electrode for all the channels.

Refractive error A defect in the ability of the lens of the eye to focus an image accurately, as occurs in nearsightedness and farsightedness.

Remuneration The amount paid to participants for their time spent in the experiment.

Rereferencing Each EEG recording has a reference electrode. For task-related EEG, the recording is linearly transformed (rereferencing) to the average of activity of all the electrodes, especially high-density EEG (>100 electrodes).

Research hypothesis A statement or proposition about the nature of the world that makes predictions about the results of an experiment. A well-formed hypothesis must be falsifiable.

Rest condition Experimental condition in which participants are not required to perform any task.

REVEAL algorithm Reverse engineering algorithm.

Sample size The selected group of participants for representation of the population.

Sample size calculation The act of choosing the number of observations or replicates to include in a statistical sample.

Scalp The skin covering the head.

Scientific evidence An empirical evidence and interpretation in accordance with scientific method that supports a scientific theory or hypothesis.

Segmentation The time-lock EEG is divided into trials, i.e., from start of trial to end, known as segmentation, to extract event-related potential (ERP) signals.

Seizure A seizure is the physical findings or changes in behavior that occur after an episode of abnormal electrical activity in the brain.

Selective serotonin reuptake inhibitors (SSRIs) A kind of drug that is typically used for treatment of major depressive disorder and anxiety.

Short-term memory The capacity of retaining, but not manipulating, a small amount of information, in the mind for a short time (less than a minute).

Signal-to-noise ratio (SNR) A measure used in signal processing and image processing that compares the level of a desired signal to the level of background noise. It is defined as the ratio of signal power to the noise power, normally expressed in decibels.

Significance level The process used by researchers to determine whether or not the null hypothesis is rejected in favor of an alternative research hypothesis.

Simulator sickness questionnaire (SSQ) This is a tool with a set of symptoms that is used in research studying simulator sickness and cyber sickness.

Standard deviation This is a quantity calculated to indicate the extent of deviation for a group as a whole in experimental data.

Statistical power The power of a statistical test is the probability that it will correctly lead to the rejection of a false null hypothesis.

Stereopsis or stereoscopic vision Vision wherein two separate images from two eyes are successfully combined into one image in the brain.

Stimulus A thing or event that evokes a specific functional reaction in an organ or tissue.

Stimulus offset The point in an EEG time series where a stimulus has ended or disappeared. It is usually described in time (milliseconds) in a time-locked EEG such as ERP signals.

Stimulus onset The point in an EEG time series where a stimulus has started or appeared. It is usually described in time (milliseconds) in a time-locked EEG such as ERP signals.

Stress condition A condition in which participants perform a cognitive task under stress environment.

Subjective assessment An assessment based on client/patient perception, understanding, and interpretation of what is happening.

Subjects rights The allowed benefits or protections to human or animal subjects in experimental research, e.g., privacy.

Synaptic transmission Synaptic transmission is a chemical event that is involved in the transmission of the impulse via release, diffusion, receptor binding of neurotransmitter molecules, and unidirectional communication between neurons.

Target population This refers to the entire group of individuals or objects to which researchers are interested in generalizing the conclusions.

Three-dimensional technology (3D) A display technology that offers the illusion of depth to the viewers.

Time-lock(ing) This is the synchronization of analysis to the events of interest that is required for extraction of epochs.

Trauma A psychologically upsetting experience that produces an emotional or mental disorder or otherwise has lasting negative effects on a person's thoughts, feelings, or behavior.

Treatment efficacy The maximum response achievable from an antidepressant; the effect of a drug.

Treatment outcome Studies undertaken to assess the results or consequences of management and procedures used in combating disease in order to determine the efficacy, effectiveness, safety, practicability, etc., of these interventions.

Trial It is also called an event. A single instance of the experimental manipulation.

T-test A statistical examination of two population means. A two-sample *t*-test examines whether two samples are different and is commonly used when the variances of two normal distributions are unknown and when an experiment uses a small sample size.

Variable A measured or manipulated quantity that changes within an experiment.

Violent games Video games that have violent content such as killing, blood, fighting, etc.

Visual discomfort The feeling of being uncomfortable while watching videos, games, or any visual stimuli, such as 3D contents.

Visual fatigue A label for conditions experienced by individuals whose work involves extended visual concentration. It describes phenomena related to intensive use of the eyes.

Visual field (VF) The area of physical space visible to an eye in a given position. The average VF is 65 degrees upward, 75 degrees downward, 60 degrees nasally, and 90 degrees temporally.

Visually induced motion sickness (VIMS) VIMS is a condition in which users of dynamic 3D contents feel symptoms of nausea, dizziness, or visual fatigue during or after exposure while they are being physically still.

Visuospatial sketchpad A component of the working memory model developed by Baddeley and Hitch in 1974. It refers to the section of one's normal mental facility that provides a virtual environment for physical simulation, calculation, visualization, and optical memory recall. It stores and processes information in a visual or spatial form.

Working memory Working memory is short-term memory. Instead of all information going into one single store, there are different systems for different types of information. It consists of a central executive that controls and coordinates the operation of two subsystems: the phonological loop and the visuospatial sketchpad.

World Health Organization The World Health Organization is a specialized agency of the United Nations that is concerned with international public health. It was established on April 7, 1948, and is headquartered in Geneva, Switzerland.

INDEX

Note: Page numbers followed by "*f*" and "*t*" refer to figures and tables, respectively.

Printed in the United States
By Bookmasters